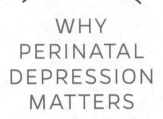

WHY
PERINATAL
DEPRESSION
MATTERS

T0151131

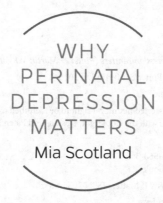

WHY
PERINATAL
DEPRESSION
MATTERS
Mia Scotland

Why Perinatal Depression Matters (Pinter & Martin Why It Matters: 4)

First published by Pinter & Martin Ltd 2015

ISBN 978-1-78066-560-3
Also available as ebook

Pinter & Martin Why It Matters ISSN 2056-8657

Series editor: Susan Last
Index: Helen Bilton
Proofreader: Debbie Kennett

British Library Cataloguing-in-Publication Data
A catalogue record for this book is available from the British Library.

Set in Minion

Printed and bound in the UK by Ashford Colour Press Ltd, Gosport, Hampshire

This book has been printed on paper that is sourced and harvested from sustainable forests and is FSC accredited.

Pinter & Martin Ltd
6 Effra Parade
London SW2 1PS

pinterandmartin.com

Contents

Generally, throughout this book, I refer to 'mother' as a biological parenting mother, and 'father' as her parenting partner who may or may not be the biological father. The content of the book is applicable in the cases where parents include adoptive mothers, or same sex couples.

'Parenthood, when it's working well, changes you. In fact, there is no change in life as great as the one you can see in a young couple, committed to each other and fully, if nervously, to starting a family.'

Steve Biddulph

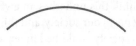

Introduction

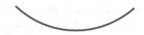

I consider myself very lucky. I have never suffered from depression. But I have studied it and tried to help others with it for over 25 years. And the more I have studied it, and worked alongside people who are suffering from it, the more thankful I become that I have never had it. I have felt pretty low sometimes. I have cried each and every day for long periods of time. I have struggled to contain my stress levels, I have been very angry and irritable, I have wished I could be more loving at times, I have thought myself to be a bad mother, and I have felt left out of things. These challenges to my mood were particularly strong after I had babies. This made sense to me. I was doing an almost impossible job, looking after two babies under 20 months old single-handedly on very little sleep. I remember curling up into a heap on the kitchen floor, crying down the phone to my beleaguered husband who was trying to do a day's work.

Looking back on this time in my life, there was actually only one thing wrong. And that was that I was on my own in the house with a little baby. All I needed was another adult around. I think this underlies an awful lot of postnatal depression problems in our society, and this book will explore some of the ways society could be kinder to mothers, fathers and babies.

I consider myself lucky because I didn't ever lose my ability to look forward to things. I didn't lose my ability to want to kiss and hold those that I loved. I didn't believe that my loved ones and my children would genuinely be better off without me in their lives. I didn't feel intense shame and confusion that I felt so bad, when I had a nice house and beautiful children. I didn't feel desperately alone and lonely even while I was surrounded by my friends and a loving husband. I didn't wake up in the morning feeling dread at the thought of getting through the day. I didn't avoid people because the effort of making conversation or saying that I was 'fine' was too great. I didn't feel like my body was a dead weight, which I had to drag through the day. I didn't feel so desperate that I would think about the only way of putting an end to it, by killing myself. I wasn't clinically depressed. My body and mind weren't shutting down.

Depression is very real. There is a myth that depression is feeling low, or that it is a case of 'mind over matter', and if people try hard enough, they can just 'snap out of it'. This might be true when we wake up feeling low. We can push on with the day until the mood lifts. But it is not true of depression. To believe that is to believe that you can 'snap out of the measles' in the same way that you can work through and ignore a mild cold.

There is also a belief that postnatal depression is somehow different from other depressions, because it is caused by hormonal fluctuations brought on by birth. The idea that women's bodies are flawed, and are the cause of their 'madness', is not new. The term 'hysteria' comes from the Latin term for 'wandering womb'. People believed that problems with women's wombs caused mental health problems. When hormones were discovered, they became the next scapegoat for women's vulnerability and fallibility. And hormones continue to be blamed for women's mood problems in adolescence, pre-menstrually throughout the woman's reproductive cycle, during pregnancy, after pregnancy, peri-menopausally and during the menopause.

But it seems we were wrong about postnatal depression. Postnatal depression is not caused by a woman's body's inability to handle hormonal fluctuations after birth. It now seems that most cases of postnatal depression actually began in pregnancy. And most people who have antenatal depression have had depression in the past. So 'postnatal depression' has now been renamed 'perinatal depression' (peri means around, as in the word 'perimeter'). It also seems that men are suffering postnatal and perinatal depression too. We haven't really been looking at this phenomenon, but the more we do, the more we see men suffering. Some studies are reporting postnatal depression rates in men to be as high as those in women. If new dads are suffering, it suggests that the problem lies in the situation, not in the body.

For some people, having a baby seems to be the straw that breaks the camel's back. Depression seems to be accounted for by the stresses that a couple experience when they have a baby. The lack of support, lack of celebration, overload of expectations, overwhelming responsibility, isolation, judgment, blaming by the media, tiredness, mixed messages, confusion, high expectations and lack of tender loving care. These stressors serve to break parents. And when we break parents, we break a baby. Babies are our future, and if we break a baby, in the long run, we break society.

Perinatal depression matters. It takes its toll on our society. It is estimated that 1 in 10 women suffer from perinatal mental health problems, and the number seems to be growing. The Royal College of Midwives found that over 25 per cent of mothers reported feeling significantly down or depressed after having their baby. It is a feminist issue, because perinatal depression is about women and their families, and valuing people, love, connection, calm and stillness over productivity, business, achievement or commerce.

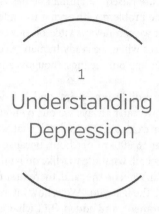

1
Understanding Depression

Depression is known as a *psychological* condition. This means that we think of depression as being something to do with our heads: our mental health, our emotions, our thoughts, our behaviours and our relationships with others. A psychologist is interested in why we do what we do, why we think what we think, and why we feel what we feel. So psychologists spend a lot of time working out why we feel depressed, how depression affects our thinking and our ability to get on with others, and how it affects what we do. We want to understand it. Get to the bottom of it. Work out how to heal people.

Psychologists are interested in what makes us all the same (common universalities of human nature, such as the need for friendship) and what makes us different to one another (such as why some people are happier in their own company than others). They are also interested in why and how we suffer (such as why some people suffer acute and chronic loneliness).

However, understanding what makes us tick is not as easy as it might seem. Understanding humans involves understanding the culture they are raised in. Human beings are a product of their culture. The problem with trying to understand human emotions, is that we can never switch off our own psychology and cultural biases when we study human psychology. So the task of understanding our feelings, thoughts and behaviours is not an easy one.

Culture is incredibly important, and it is what shapes us as humans, but we can't always *see* our own culture, because we are in it. For example, we can't tell that we are spinning through space at 16,000km per hour, because we are *in it*. A fish once asked a crab what life was like on land. The crab said, 'It's sandy, you can walk on the sand, there's a sun in the sky and there's no water'. The fish said, 'Wow, how interesting'. Then he thought for a moment, and added, 'But what is water?' Freud famously spent years puzzling over the question 'What *does* a woman want?' He couldn't fathom why women seemed so lost, restless, unhappy and anxious. He couldn't see that ladies needed more than polite society. He literally could not see what seems so obvious to us now, that his society treated women as second-rate citizens, inferior physically and mentally, and that this affected their emotional wellbeing. Freud was astute and he did think outside the box, but he never did manage to understand that women were reacting to a society which was not able to meet their needs. Women, like men, need exercise, respect, challenges, equality, and broader role definitions. He was trapped in a culture that regarded women as creatures who just needed to rest in their vulnerability and delicate frames, or their mental health would be compromised and they would get a 'wandering womb' in the form of hysteria.

Another reason that understanding human emotion, including depression, is difficult, is because our society has presumed for many years that the psychological and the physical are separate entities. Ever since the philosopher

Descartes cemented the growing notion that mind and body are separate in the 1600s, we in the West have used language, made presumptions and behaved in a way that presumes this dualism to be true. Depression comes under the umbrella of 'psychological' or 'emotional' or 'in the mind'. However, recent research is challenging this notion that mind and body can be separated. For example, we are beginning to understand that the experience of physical pain is not physical *or* mental, it is both. It is a combination of the two. We are learning that 'physical' conditions have a strong psychological component, including cancer, heart disease and diabetes. Seemingly 'psychological' conditions can also have a very physical component, such as depression associated with wheat intolerance. The placebo effect is regarded as 'in the mind', but how can this be? The whole point of the placebo effect is that it directly impacts on our physical body, creating very real changes in the form of healing (or in the case of the nocebo effect, creating illness in the body). The dualism between mind and body has led to a complete overlooking of the fact that placebo is a *physical* healer of illness. When trying to understand depression, I would urge us to move away from the notion that it is a psychological condition. It is not. It is a human condition, wrapped up in our crazy, amazing bodies, and in our unique and bizarre culture.

Thus, the mind and the body cannot be separated. Really understanding this will go a long way to lifting the stigma that is attached to mental health problems. The individual and society cannot be separated either. Society builds individuals, and we are all a product of our society. A human being cannot survive without society (we know that babies die if they don't receive social interaction).

In trying to understand depression, we need to understand our society. We need to understand what kind of mothers, fathers, and babies, our society is building. Only then can we shed some light on why so many mothers and fathers seem to be struggling with perinatal depression.

Society's messages – is motherhood blissful, or is it awful?

When you think of motherhood, what do you envisage? As a young woman studying feminism in the 1980s, I was sold the idea that motherhood is a thankless, down-trodden, boring task. I was told that the word 'housewife' was demeaning. I was taught that if I had children, I would lose my identity, I would become 'just' a mother, and my career, my individuality, my spark and my independence would be taken from me. People would look down on me. I would become used and reduced to domesticity. I was taught that the 'myth' of blissful motherhood is peddled by a society that wants to enchain women into the slavery that is motherhood. I was taught that people who believed in blissful mothering were being sold a lie, and that it was just a tool of social control to keep women chained to the kitchen sink.

The opposing view of motherhood is that it is blissful. Motherhood is the ultimate goal in a female's life – her evolutionary biology is geared to find fulfilment in becoming a mother, and that is all she needs, because that is so rewarding in and of itself. Once she births a baby, and falls in love with it, she finds joy, and fulfilment. She needs nothing more, but to love and devote her time to her baby. She will find this easy and joyful, because it comes naturally to her. This view of motherhood is exemplified by the popularity of natural birth movements, extolling the joy of ecstatic birthing hormones and orgasmic birth. If formula advertising wasn't so successful, I daresay it would be more mainstream to extol the joys of breastfeeding, idealising the ecstatic, warming bond that mother and baby feel as they connect in a swirl of oxytocined-up loveliness.

I don't know about you, but I find these stereotypes very unhelpful. I'm not saying that they aren't true, because there is some truth in each of them. The problem is that they are unrealistically black and white, and leave parents feeling inadequate (because they aren't ecstatic) or uneasy (expecting the job to be so unfulfilling).

If you think these stereotypes aren't prevalent, or you think I'm exaggerating, think again. They are part of our society, and they underpin all that we do – our presumptions, our habits and practices, and our legislation. Examples are everywhere. Providing free nursery places so that women can get back to being 'productive'. Thinking it is okay to leave new mums alone at home weeks after they've had the baby, because mothering is natural and easy. I've heard fathers use the excuse 'You're naturally more patient with the baby than me' to get out of looking after their own children. I've heard women say, time and time again, 'Why am I finding this so difficult when it comes naturally to others?', and feel guilty and inadequate because they didn't fall in love with their baby straight away.

Conversely, women return to work six weeks after having baby because they believe that being 'just' a stay-at-home mum isn't enough for them. Women go back to work so they can feel that they are 'providing' for the family, because 'just' being at home with the children doesn't count. And so on. The myths are damaging because they contribute to the rates and severity of postnatal depression in women. In not valuing motherhood, in not helping women meet their biological needs, in not giving women the time, respect and care that they need to become happy, proud, competent mothers, we risk increasing postnatal depression.

Society needs to allow a woman to develop slowly and fully as a mother, not to view birth as a one off 'event', in which she went from a 'non-mother' to 'a mother' in six hours of labour, suddenly equipped and good to go. We need to value and respect the enormous energy that goes into creating a new mother. While the feminism that I was raised with tended to ignore motherhood, there is a new wave of feminism that attends to motherhood, and tries to understand and celebrate it. As Maddie McMahon, doula and feminist, puts it, using the three-day blues as an example, 'The day three blues will continue if we don't know how our bodies work and what makes our babies and boobs so damn magical. When no one's given us permission to love the *process* of mothering, we forget the joy and just focus on the worries that we are doing everything wrong'.

As a culture, we need to be working together to help the mother grow into a mother. Viewing motherhood as a delicate process that requires the attention of all those around her (the father, her close family, her extended family, health care professionals, her employers) is something that our society does not do, at a cost to her health. Let's take a look now at how our society differs from others around the globe, and you'll see what I mean.

Care of mothers in other societies

Many cultures across time and space share a similar form of behaviour. They have inbuilt cultural norms which involve *stopping the new mother from doing very much at all* after she has had her baby. The length of time that this goes on for is oddly similar in all these cultures. It lasts approximately forty days or six weeks. This practice is so common in other cultures that modern Western culture seems to be the odd one out.

How, as a culture, do we do postnatal care in Great Britain? Mothers generally give birth in a hospital. About thirty years ago, it was expected that mum would stay in a hospital bed for about two weeks, before going home with her baby. Nowadays, mothers are told they can go home six hours after giving birth. This suits the hospitals (which are struggling to cope with the demands that a postnatal ward makes on staffing levels). It also suits the women, who often *really* want to get home as soon as possible. We sort of accept this: of course you want to get home to your own house, your own things, and your own partner.

But the issue of women wanting to get home as quickly as possible needs to be explored a little more. Why do they want to go home so soon? Researchers have found that mothers are eager to go home early due to a perceived lack of support from midwives on the postnatal ward (Ockleford et al, 2004). Julie Wray found that women were much more satisfied with their postnatal care outside of hospital, than they were with their care inside hospital. The areas they found wanting included cleanliness, visiting arrangements, noise, rest and support for infant feeding and baby care. If women felt cared for, safe, nurtured and comfortable in hospital, would they really want to go home as soon as possible? If their partners could stay with them in the room, would they want to go home as soon as possible? If they had a choice of delicious, nutritious food, would they really want to go home as soon as possible? If they could get a good night's sleep, would they really want to go home? If there was compassionate and skilled advice and support available in hospital (including feeding, bathing, looking after the cord, how to change the baby and keep the baby warm), would women be as keen to get home? A woman with a new baby needs all of these things. She needs comfort, good food, help with caring for the baby and people she loves around her. If she can't get that in hospital, it stands to reason that she will want to go home.

Given that women in our culture generally return home quite soon after having a baby, what support systems are in place to help her settle in and adapt to life as a mother, with a new baby? Often the father brings them home. Sometimes, they come back to an empty house. Often the father will have a week or two of leave from work to help settle in with the baby. It is common to have arranged for a grandmother to come and stay for a week or so, to help with household chores and food preparation. They will have some follow-up visits from health workers or appointments at a clinic to have the baby weighed and 'check' that all is going well. The mother will have been advised to 'leave the housework, grab sleep while you can, and don't accept too many visitors'. But if she is going to 'leave the housework', who is going to do it instead? If she doesn't manage to 'grab sleep' while she can, what does she do then? And how does she feel when she has visitors that stayed a lot longer than she had agreed that they would? Is that her fault? Not only is she expected to manage her own time, her visitors, and her ability to learn to live in a dirty, messy house, but she is also being subtly blamed for not getting it right, if she is stressed about the house or taking too many visitors.

The postnatal period is thus full of promise, but can involve much more than the new parents bargained for. They can't wait to get away from the hospital, to get home, to be together with their baby, to show their baby off to visitors and to 'play house' together. But when they get home, the reality can be very different. They have started a full-time, 24-hour job which they were not trained for. They have to start the job suffering from lack of sleep, feeling tired and overwhelmed. They realise the impact of not being able to rest, or think, or regroup emotionally. They feel physically exhausted, emotionally drained and overwhelmed very quickly indeed. In the meantime, the house is getting messier and messier, and dirtier and dirtier, and the baby cries way more than they had realised, and they didn't anticipate the endless, dark, long and lonely nights.

Other cultures do things differently. They don't send a

couple home alone and expect them to manage the house, the food, the visitors and the long dark nights on their own.

Japan

'In the Japanese islands of the Goto Archipelago… a new mother is expected to stay in bed, wrapped in her quilt, for one month after delivery. Her baby is wrapped up next to her. Grandmothers, aunts, and relatives come in to take care of her, feeding her and helping her to the bathroom. She is expected to do nothing but feed her baby and recover. While her relatives help her, they speak to her in a form of baby talk. In response, she answers them in a high-pitched voice. For one month, she is a child in their eyes. A postpartum recovery period is accepted and treated as normal in this culture.' (taken from Brazelton, 2006). Indeed, across Japan as a whole, the postnatal period is given due reverence and is known as 'satogaeri'. This tradition ensures that the mother gets plenty of rest, and adjusts to her new life and her new baby.

India

In India, the first forty days after birth are also seen as a 'confinement' period, when the mother is given time and space to recuperate, gain strength and bond with her new baby. Nutritious food is an important part of this tradition, and each region of India has its own favourite postnatal foods that the mother is given. In some areas of India, the new mother is given a full body massage, or maalish, once a day. Imagine how that would feel! Being given special home-cooked food each day, and a full body massage. Bliss.

Hispanic countries

In Hispanic countries, similar reverence and importance is given to the postnatal period. They have a wonderful tradition for new mothers, known as *la cuarentena*, which is still practised in many countries. This is a period of approximately forty days, or six weeks, during which the new mother abstains from sex and is solely dedicated to breastfeeding and taking care of her baby and herself. During this time, other members of the family pitch in to cook, clean, and take care of other children, if there are any. In some Latin American countries it's traditional to use herbal remedies during this period to aid in recovery. It's also common to offer the new mother special meals, such as vegetable soups made from scratch. Once this period is over, it's believed, the new mother is ready to return in full to family life.

Malaysia

In Malaysia, the confinement period is known as a *pantang*, which lasts about forty-four days. It is designed to preserve the health and femininity of the mother. She receives hot stone massages to cleanse the womb and a full-body exfoliation treatment said to smooth, soften and lighten the skin, chasing away postpartum body changes. New mothers are not allowed to lift heavy things or do anything apart from nursing the baby. All of the house chores fall to the husband, relatives who volunteer, or a hired helper. Try to imagine how incredibly healing this would be – good food, lots of rest and relaxation, regular hot stone massages and a full-body exfoliation treatment!

In the UK, it seems to me that there is only one way that we have of really honouring the mother when she gets home. And that is to bring a present and a congratulations card. Some people may bring food, and some may offer to help. Family might come to help for a week or two. But the mother will often find herself getting out of bed, doing the school run, cleaning, making herself a sandwich, showering on her own, cleaning the toilet and so on. She is expected to get back to 'normal' as soon as possible, which includes getting back to her pre-pregnancy weight and shape. It is no wonder that some women are left feeling low, overwhelmed, run down, poorly and depressed.

I know that there is a counter-argument to this. I know that many people will argue with me, and say 'But women *want* to get back into a routine, they don't *want* to lie in bed for four weeks, they'd go crazy, they want to get out and about again as soon as possible'. And that is what is wrong with our culture. We do not understand that a new mother is just that. New. She needs to recover, learn and adapt, and that takes time. Things can't be the same again. Her body *has* changed forever. Her mind and soul *are* different. She has to find strength, knowledge and power to be this thing that is a mother. Being a mother is different from being a housekeeper or employee. A mother needs to be emotionally present. A mother of a baby needs to live life at a slower pace. She needs to be instantly interruptible. She needs to have a body that can heal, and produce milk. She needs to get used to never really finishing or achieving anything. She can't go back to her old life. She can't be active, busy and slim if she is to adjust effectively to having a new baby in her life.

There is an awful lot going on for the mother and father as they recover from birth and adapt to life with a new baby. That is why these other cultures take the postnatal recovery and adaptation period so seriously. They have done this intuitively. Research is beginning to show that they were right. When you begin to understand the changes that are actually going on for the mother and baby during the postnatal time, we can see why loving care of the mother is so important.

Physical adjustment during the postnatal period

I have separated physical adjustment from emotional adjustment because that is how our language and thinking works. There are not the words to explain perinatal adjustment as a systemic, whole-body process. However, although I talk about them separately, this is not to say that one does not affect the other. We know, with increasing confidence, that when you look after yourself physically, this impacts on your endocrine system, your nervous system and your neurological system (in other words, your emotional health). Likewise, if you take care of your emotional needs, this impacts on your immune system and your cardiovascular system (in other words, your physical health).

Do not underestimate what your body needs to do after you have had a baby. Your body is an incredible machine, which managed to *grow a whole human being* on its own. It then managed to go through the actual birth: whether you did it entirely on your own, or with some hospital intervention, or with a caesarean section, your body went through changes to get that baby out. It went through quite a process! And it needs to make changes, adapt and recover as a result. Research suggests that this takes more than a few days in hospital and a few more at home. It takes between six weeks and a whole year.

The uterus is shrinking back down in size, which involves further contractions, and lochia – vaginal bleeding that can continue for up to six weeks. If you do too much physically, then the bleeding may be heavier or last longer.

All the organs in your body that were scrunched up when your baby was inside, slowly move back to where they came from, including the muscles in the abdomen, which need to come together again slowly to prevent ongoing separation.

You are establishing breastfeeding, which is a magnificent hormonal, physiological, psychological and physical process that takes up to 500 extra calories a day. Also, successful breastfeeding relies on the production of oxytocin, which will not be produced easily if the mother is stressed or anxious. At the beginning, breastfeeding can be sore, and the body needs to stay healthy to avoid problems such as infections, mastitis or thrush.

If you are not establishing breastfeeding, then your body is adapting to the changes needed to stop the milk flow, which may lead to tenderness and discomfort due to engorgement.

If you have had a perineal tear or some form of intervention (such as an assisted birth or a caesarean section) there is tissue damage which also needs to heal. Your body has an injury, and it needs rest and good food to help it to do so smoothly and free of infection.

You are recovering physically from the act of birth itself, which, at the very least, probably meant that you lost out on some sleep. Lack of sleep is not conducive to good physical recovery, because it is while we sleep that the body goes about restoring and replenishing tissue damage and fighting infection.

Your body is making some crazy hormonal changes to adjust and adapt to you not being pregnant any more. These impact on your mood, your appetite, your need for love, peace, sleep and relaxation. It even impacts on your hair growth!

What makes for a good physical recovery?

There are the obvious things that help us to recover more quickly, and we all know about them. In our 'go-getting' society, we often ignore them, prioritising being busy and achieving over activities such as resting and eating good food. It makes sense that most traditions emphasise feeding the mother and keeping her in bed while other people do the chores. But did you know that care and compassion also help you to heal? This is because the body releases oxytocin in response to feeling loved. Oxytocin is a hormone of healthy cell growth and wound healing. The hormones that temporarily inhibit healing and growth are stress hormones, such as adrenalin and cortisol. It is really important that a new mother worries as little as possible. We don't want her to be worrying about getting things wrong, or feeling like a failure, or concerned about looking after visitors, or stressed that her body looks flabby and fat, or having to cope with a crying baby on her own at night, or any of the many pressures that are on new mothers in our society. On the contrary, we want her to feel epic, special, nurtured and proud. And I'm not just saying this because I'm a wannabe do-gooder who likes candles and tree hugging. I'm saying this because if we don't, we risk having new mothers who are not able to recover physically from birth. Other societies seem to have understood this at an intuitive level. Why not us?

As well as recovering physically from birth, there are a few more challenges for your mind and body during the postnatal period.

Emotional adjustment during the postnatal period

A mother is not just a vessel for growing and birthing a baby. Once she has had the baby, we aren't left with an 'un-pregnant woman' and a baby. We have a mother and a baby. This mother needs to adapt to her new life, and adapt to her baby, if she is to take on the role of feeding, physically caring for, and emotionally responding to her baby.

Adjustment to immobility

One of the many jobs that a new mother needs to adapt to is being relatively immobile. As a breastfeeding mother in particular, you will need to sit regularly for many hours continuously. This may be very different to your pre-mother life. You may have been very active, energetic and busy. Even if you are not breastfeeding, you will not be able to dart in and out of the house, because getting out of the house with a baby can take a very long time.

Adjustment to being instantly interruptible

As a new mother, you need to be able to respond to your

baby's needs instantly. You can't ask a baby to wait. A crying baby is one of the most stressful sounds a mother can endure (this makes sense, as we know from research that to leave a baby crying is not healthy for the baby, so mothers have been evolutionarily programmed to want to stop babies from crying). Your baby needs you to be able to drop whatever you are doing so that you can respond to their needs. You cannot decide to wait ten minutes while you finish your email.

Adjustment to being responsible

As a new mother, you are responsible for the life of another being for the first time in your life. If we lived in communities with wise and experienced family around, this would not be such a big issue, and most mothers would probably not even notice it. Everyone is responsible for keeping the baby alive, and those who have done it before are pretty relaxed about the whole process, which helps you to relax. But in our culture, the mother and the father often come home to an empty house with a brand new baby to *keep alive* on their own! They have never done this before, and they can feel overwhelmed by the sense of responsibility.

Adjustment to slowing down

Everything happens very slowly with a baby around. Feeding can take hours, getting out of the house can take hours, getting dressed can take hours. If you're in a rush, this is going to lead to frustration and stress, which is not helpful for the parents or for the baby. So learning to slow down can be a major adjustment for some new parents.

Adjustment to loss of routine

Before you had your baby, you might have tended to shower first thing, head down for breakfast, have a cup of tea before your cereal, put your make-up on, pack your bag, and grab your coat. You may not have realised how important this routine was to you, having done it for the majority of your adult life. When a baby comes along, the routine becomes impossible. I remember struggling to get used to packing my baby bag before eating breakfast. It just felt wrong, but I soon learned that if I didn't do it, I would never get out of the house. I also struggled with not showering until the evening, and having to go some days without showering. This is a process of adjustment. An experienced mother will have no problems making these adjustments, and will think nothing of it. A new mother is more likely to feel lost, frustrated, resentful and/or stressed.

Adjustment to not putting yourself first

Throughout your life, to some extent, you have been able to put yourself first. When a baby comes along, your needs come second to the baby's. You are hungry – you have just made a delicious-looking sandwich – but the baby wakes up, and you have to leave your sandwich until later. You are tired, you need to sleep, you have just dropped off to sleep… and the baby wakes. You cannot sleep until later. You are ill, and you need to go to bed for a day, but your baby needs you to be up and about, responding to her needs. The hormone prolactin, known as the motherhood hormone because it is involved with lactation, helps a mother to be more submissive and to put her baby's needs before her own. It is an important part of adjusting to motherhood.

Adjustment to not being able to focus on a task

Ever since our school days, we have been encouraged to focus on one task at a time, and to finish tasks that we have started. Being told to 'concentrate, don't talk while working, don't start another game until you've put the last one away, a job isn't done until you've cleared away, finish the assignment by Friday' has helped us to be productive students, employees and housekeepers. However, when a baby comes along, the ability to focus on one task and see it through to the end becomes academic. It simply isn't possible. A new parent needs to multi-task, be constantly interrupted and have no hope of finishing anything, not even a cup of tea. This takes quite some adjustment, and can involve a good deal of frustration and stress, particularly if you have achieved a lot of qualifications and had a successful career.

Making the most of adjusting to parenthood

The process of becoming a parent is just that – a process. It is not a one-off biological event, after which a mother can get back to normal. If we are to respect our biology, it would seem that becoming a mother is a developmental process which takes time to flourish and develop, both physically and psychologically. As parenting author Steve Biddulph puts it 'the shift that comes about in early parenthood, and then ripens and increases with great rewards as the years speed by, is to learn about the joy – and freedom – of not being self-focused'. We don't learn this in one night. We begin the adventurous journey with birth, which is 'a kind of baptism of fire… we are exploded into that sense of being on a rollercoaster or surfing on a huge wave, where we can steer and balance but we can never completely control the massive forces of life that carry us along'. In order to help her adjust, the mother needs to have stresses and strains removed. Slowing down, recovering and adjusting takes time. Added to this, arguably, the most important adjustment that the mother needs to make is to bond with her baby.

Pregnancy matters too

Postnatal depression has been renamed perinatal depression. This is because research has shown us that most cases of postnatal depression actually start in pregnancy. This is important information, because it means that if a woman is depressed during pregnancy, she needs extra special care, because there is an increased chance that she will struggle even more after the baby is born. If you are depressed during your pregnancy, then it is great that you are reading this book, because you need to take your needs seriously, listen to your body and mind, and begin to prepare now for making the baby phase as smooth as it can be.

Is this new information, which we didn't previously know? Research is only as good as the questions that it asks, and if research never bothered to ask women 'Were you depressed during your pregnancy?' then we might never have known. Or could it be that things changed? Could it be that mothers and fathers didn't used to become stressed and depressed in pregnancy, to the extent that they do now? Could things have changed, to make pregnancy more stressful and depressing than it used to be? I think the answer is yes.

In our modern technology-ridden lives, we are constantly plugged into a stream of information from the television, from magazines, and from social media. This is creating an epidemic of stress and depression. There is simply so much information out there about what might harm your baby, that I'm surprised anyone makes it through a pregnancy without feeling incredibly vulnerable and as though they are walking on eggshells. We are so bombarded with conflicting advice, warnings and scare stories that our brains are constantly getting the message that 'it is dangerous and precarious to be pregnant, you could very easily do something wrong, and your body will let you down at any moment'. Even the 'reassuring' custom of having a scan actually implies that your baby needs to be 'checked' because something might be wrong. I didn't enjoy the journey to the hospital, the waiting-rooms, the form-filling, checking the sonographer's face to see that she was staying relaxed… If the 'results' come back unclear, that can send a couple into a tailspin of frantic anxiety, often needlessly. The NHS runs on a 'better safe than sorry' system. I'm not saying it shouldn't be like that, but I am saying that this leads to a lot of false positive 'results' and a lot of emotional fall-out.

Emotional fall-out matters in pregnancy, because the emotional care that the mother is given reaps rewards for the developing baby. Science is revealing a great deal about the emotional health of the mother in pregnancy, and the benefits of taking extra special care of the mother to reduce her stress levels. We know that mother-baby bonding begins in pregnancy, and if we promote that in the form of classes and workshops, the benefits for the baby last *at least* six years (on average, statistically speaking). We know that if you furnish a mother with a relaxation CD during her pregnancy, you directly reduce her fear of birth. That matters, because if she is less frightened of the birth, she can relax better in her pregnancy, and relaxation in pregnancy matters because it builds a better brain for the baby (generally speaking). We know that if a mother can bond with her baby and create a 'secure attachment relationship' with her baby, the benefits for the baby last a lifetime. This information is statistically gathered, so it doesn't actually tell us anything about you as an individual, because your life will be full of all sorts of other factors that change the picture. However, it does tell us something about what our culture could do to enhance the health of the growing baby.

According to the research, there is one thing that society could do to enhance the health of our nation: take care of the mother's emotional wellbeing during pregnancy. There are many ways a government might address this (for example, ensuring that Surestart services remain well-funded, increasing maternity leave before birth as well as after birth, enhancing compassionate midwifery care, addressing social inequality and so on). However, the purpose of this book isn't to advise government. It is to advise you. Take your pregnancy seriously. Pregnancy is a time to take stock and review your life habits. Try to avoid cramming everything in before baby arrives. On the contrary, begin to slow down and take care of yourself. Allow others to help you, give yourself permission to nurture yourself and reduce the number of very stressful things in your life. (Stress comes in many forms, and everyone needs a bit of stress to function well. Boredom can be as stressful as being busy.)

A great deal of this book applies to pregnancy as well as the time after your baby has been born – the whole perinatal period. Your baby's brain is growing and developing during pregnancy as well as after birth. Your hormonal and neurological system is changing and adapting, and you are bonding with your baby, although you might not be aware of that. All the other chapters that look at how to avoid depression taking hold, and how to manage it if you do become depressed, also apply to the pregnancy stage of your journey to parenthood, as well as after the birth of your baby.

A word about research, statistics and evidence

Research is important for helping us sift out what is actually good for us, and what isn't. It helped us understand just how bad smoking is for our health. However, research can scare us, and it can be misleading. It can be misleading for too many reasons to list here, but one reason is that research is only interested in very large numbers of people. It is not interested in individuals like you or me. If you read somewhere that research shows that eating crisps is bad for you, you may feel bad when you eat a packet of crisps. If you have eaten lots of crisps, or given your child lots of crisps, you may feel even worse. But research over-generalises, and over-simplifies, and ignores other important aspects of our lives. Research tells us about generalities, but nothing about ourselves as individuals. For example, if a study found that eating crisps is bad for you, this does not mean that *you* will be unhealthy if you eat crisps. It only tells us that generally, in a huge sample of people, there are more unhealthy people among those that eat crisps, compared with those that don't. This difference is probably very small, which is why research needs big samples of people before the differences can even be noticed. In other words, many people who eat crisps are healthy, and many people who don't eat crisps are not healthy. But the group of people who eat crisps *and* are unhealthy is slightly bigger. We know, in general, that people who eat crisps are less healthy, but it does not tell us anything about *you*, because you don't know which of these circles you fit into, if you eat crisps. We also don't

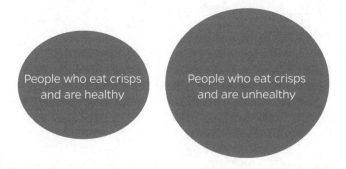

know how many crisps *you* need to eat to see an effect on your health. Neither do we know how much other health-giving aspects of your life may mitigate against the negative effects of crisp-eating, such as loving, laughing, exercising, relaxing, taking vitamins, eating roughage and so on.

Thus, although we know that eating crisps isn't good for us, we also know that the body is very good at processing junk food and getting rid of it, and that nothing bad will happen if you eat crisps. This is the same as knowing that tall people bang their heads more – but it doesn't mean that all tall people always bang their heads, and it doesn't mean that short people don't bang their heads, and it doesn't mean that tall people don't have great ways of adapting to their height. It's the same for you and your baby. Although I do quote research here and there, I want you to remember that research is very general, and tells us very little about you as a complicated individual with so much other stuff going on in your life.

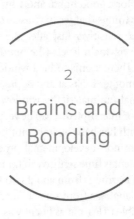

2

Brains and
Bonding

The connection between a mother or father and their baby is a strong one. We all want beautiful, healthy babies. But more than that, evolution has equipped us with a need for *our own* baby. If a hospital were to say that they aren't sure which baby is yours (as they got a bit mixed up in the nursery), but that they have given you the prettiest and healthiest baby by far, you would not be impressed. Nature has designed us to want to invest in our own babies, and it has designed us to be rather good at putting our own babies first. This ensures the baby gets the love and nurturing that it needs. The process that helps us do this is a biological evolutionary mechanism. It is 'bonding', and it is apparent in all mammals. In some rather tragic cases, the process doesn't work. For example, ewes will now and again reject their lambs, and not have anything to do with them. But most tragically, the bonding process can go wrong in humans. I have often heard mothers say 'I feel like I am just going through the motions. I'm just looking after a baby, because I have to, but it could be anybody's baby'. While we have an awful lot to learn about what makes for a good bond, and why it sometimes goes wrong, there a few things that we have ascertained.

Bonding is time sensitive. Just after the baby is born, the mother and baby's oxytocin levels (the bonding hormone) are very high indeed. There seems to be a window of opportunity, during which the mother looks at and *begins* to fall in love with her baby. In mammals/animals, if this window of opportunity for bonding is missed or interrupted, it can be very difficult to get the mother to bond with her baby at any point in the future. 'Time sensitivity' is a common developmental process. For example, language development is time sensitive in humans. If we miss the natural window of learning (from about two to eight years old), and try to learn a language from scratch later on, it can be very difficult or impossible to learn it as fluently as a child can.

With birth and bonding in humans, if the process is disrupted just after birth and the window of opportunity is missed, we don't really know what the implications are. We do know that mothers and babies can and do bond very effectively, but it seems that the process can be longer and slower if they miss the opportunity directly after birth. The bonding process is brought about by touch, smell, fondling, holding, massaging, looking, eye contact and so on. Oxytocin is the hormone that brings this about, and it is mediated by quiet, warmth and a feeling of safety. In animals, we know that if we disturb or upset the mother during this process, there is a danger of disrupting the bonding process by disturbing the production of oxytocin. So in theory, if we disturb or upset a human mother, we also interrupt her natural flow of oxytocin, which might disrupt her ability to fall in love with her baby.

To thrive or to survive – the baby brain decides

During the process of evolution, our minds and bodies have become very good at making sure we stay alive.

We automatically notice and respond to danger in our environment. We have very finely tuned and efficient survival instincts, which operate almost on a moment to moment basis. For example, if I suddenly hear a noise while I am writing this book, my immediate reaction will be hypervigilance and alertness. I look up, my heart races a little, I might even jump out of my skin. This all happens in a split second, before I have even had time to think 'What is that noise?' Survival instincts in humans are the *first* port of call. They take priority over everything else, because if we hadn't managed to stay alive, there'd be no chance to get anything else right in life. Staying alive comes before enjoyment. We need to be alive, before we can thrive. But if we have no worries about staying alive, if we are basically safe, and don't need to worry too much about surviving, we can then begin to thrive.

Babies have the same issues. If they are in an environment that is basically safe, they can begin to thrive. They can relax, look around a lot, smile at adults, learn and take in their surroundings, and their brains will adapt accordingly, and 'fire and wire' the relevant neural connections. If they are in an environment that doesn't feel all that safe, they need to activate their 'stay alive' mechanisms, in the form of crying or shutting down or staying hyper-vigilant. These behaviours are mediated via the production of the stress hormones cortisol and adrenalin. So in an environment where the baby cries, and is responded to quickly, they are getting the message 'I'm protected by an adult, I'm safe'. The baby relaxes, which is mediated by the production of oxytocin, among other hormones. Conversely, if the baby cries and there is no response, the baby might respond as if to say 'Where is the person that keeps me alive? Why are they not responding to me? What is wrong?' At that point, the baby may stop crying temporarily (not to stop the metaphorical wolf from finding them, but to give mum time to look for where the cry came from) or they may increase their distress signal, and cry harder or begin to scream. This increases their stress hormone levels. As stress hormone levels increase, the baby's brain 'wires and fires' the parts of the brain associated with staying vigilant and alert to danger. (Please remember, when reading this, that some stress is good for all of us, even babies, and that all babies cry to differing degrees, just like all adults moan or laugh to differing degrees.)

The parent/baby relationship – growing a healthy brain

When a stranger comes up to a baby in a pram, what is the first thing that they usually do? Typically, they put on a great big smile, lean down to look at the baby, and make strong 'cooing' noises. (Or is that just me?) The baby usually responds with a great big grin. This grin reinforces the adult's behaviour; they laugh in delight and coo and smile even more. Delight and joy are shared between baby and adult. Research in brain-imaging is beginning to show us that this interaction is very important and health-giving for the baby. It creates a myriad of neuronal activity in the brain, activating certain parts and helping the baby brain to grow (after babies are born, brain growth continues, particularly in the first two years of life). The healthy brain growth that comes with reciprocal joy and social interaction happens largely in the pre-frontal cortex, which is associated with regulation of stress and emotion. So the more interactive play and joy that a baby receives, the more the brain responds with healthy neuronal growth. As Sue Gerhardt puts it 'love drives the development of the brain'. Prolonged and/or repeated severe stress does the opposite, and can inhibit healthy growth of the brain. If the mother (or other caretaker) has bonded well with her baby, enjoys her baby, and can be pretty calm and attentive to her baby, then the baby has more chance of learning to relax, enjoy life, and thrive.

Thus the neural growth of a baby's brain seems to happen in an adaptive, healthy way when there is the feeling of joy and relaxation in the baby's environment. Joy and relaxation are the antidote to stress. No one feels joy or relaxation when there is a metaphorical 'tiger in the bushes'. And here we have the problem with depression. Depression makes us joyless. And it also makes us stressed. So when babies are in an environment where there is only one main carer in the house, day in day out, and when that main carer is depressed, the baby is more likely to activate the 'survive' button than the 'thrive' button. Research suggests that this can have consequences for the baby's ability to get on with others in later life, their ability to manage stress and their chances of getting depression. We know that stress and depression in mothers is not good for them or their babies. Of course, this is statistically speaking. I want you to remember that each individual is very complex, and very resourceful.

Mothers grow bigger brains too

New mothers are not just vessels from which a baby has popped, and then the mother returns to how she was before. Oh no. She is now a mother. This involves a fair amount of transition: hormonally, physiologically, physically, neuro-biologically and psychologically. She experiences a well of feelings that she may never have had before, such as a fierce sense of protection for the infant, or a deep love that is different to any she has felt before. The intensity of breastmilk beginning to flow, the love for others around her, the exhaustion of lack of sleep, the overwhelming sense of responsibility, the soreness of stretched and tired muscles.

Although our society is embracing equality and blurring of the gendered stereotypes of our forefathers, we must not underestimate the enormity of the fact that a mother grows and births her baby, and breastfeeds the baby. Her body is designed to do this, and doing it involves a fair amount of magical work from her biological, hormonal, physiological and neurological systems. In orchestrating all these adaptations and changes, the mother's brain also undergoes dramatic changes. As she releases oxytocin and prolactin in response to breastfeeding, her body responds with increased trust, love, passivity, reduced stress response, reduced restlessness and increased submissiveness. The brain responds neurologically, and although science is only just beginning to explore this in humans, it seems that her brain actually grows in response to the changing demands of motherhood.

Brain growth is optimised by joy and calm. The calmer the environment for the mother, the more likely nature's orchestration is to unfold optimally. In my view, this may be a time sensitive process. It may be that if we miss the window of opportunity for helping the mother settle into her new role, she might not fully establish those feelings that come with the heady mix of prolactin and oxytocin, such as increased trust, love, passivity and submissiveness that we see in other mammals. Research has not yet asked this question.

We all need to take extra special care of mothers

So it seems that warm, positive, joyful interaction between mother and baby is optimal in regulating the baby's development of the immune system and stress response. A good bond and a relaxed mother both help with this process. I don't mean that the mother needs to do her best to relax and enjoy her baby. I mean that everybody else should take care of the mother, so that she can enjoy her baby. The very act of 'needing' to relax stops one from being able to relax. You can't be 'instructed' to enjoy something, or 'try'. That is about as useful as telling someone to relax while watching a horror movie or they will have a heart attack. Enjoyment and relaxation is a state of being, not an action. It takes a village to raise a child. A mother cannot be solely responsible for the welfare of herself, the baby, her finances, the house, and stay sane. She needs support from others to be able to enjoy motherhood.

This is a feminist issue which feminism has, until recently, failed to address. The pervasive issues around not valuing femininity for fear of viewing it as biological destiny, or being concerned with being 'equal' to men, as opposed to different but equally valued, have, I believe, taken us to a place where the job of being a mother, and all that it entails, and the high status that should accompany it, have only just begun to be addressed by feminist thinkers. We lack the genuine respect for the work that mothers do, we throw angry insults at them for 'choosing' to become mothers, we ignore that they might be lonely, isolated or struggling when the baby arrives, we disregard their bad birth experiences because 'Oh well, at least you have a healthy baby' and so on. Raising children is a big deal. If we raise them well, we pre-empt many problems in society, such as delinquency, aggression, learning difficulties, additional needs, mental health problems, workforce issues, and so on. Get the parenting right, and we get such a lot of other things right too.

You might be thinking that I should be writing about 'parents' a little more, and writing about 'mothers' a little less. While society is breaking down the gender stereotypes reassuringly fast, I think there is now a danger of subsuming motherhood into 'parenthood' and thereby losing what is special about mothers. Don't get me wrong, dads do matter, dads do make great parents, and there are many single fathers and two-dad families out there. Separated dads have access rights and so they should. But dads are different. They really are! Mothers and fathers are not the same. They look very different because they have adapted to fulfil differing evolutionary functions. Their bodies look different, and I suspect their brains are also different.

We seem to be intent on blurring the sexes, carrying on one of the mistakes that feminism made during the 1970s. Mothers gestate and carry the baby for nine months. Fathers do not. Mothers, and only mothers, birth their babies. Mothers, and only mothers, breastfeed their babies. Mothers evolved to do all those things perfectly well, just as every other mammal on the planet has. Mothers are evolved to instantly protect their baby at birth. They are equipped for it, with their wombs, their breasts, their hips, their brains, their endocrine systems and so on. They are special in their own way. It might sound old-fashioned, but I think that mothers need to identify what makes them feminine, so they can be proud of that, in the same way that fathers need to be proud of their masculinity. Chapter 4, about dads, suggests that societal changes are moving at such a pace that men are in the midst of a great deal of confusion about what it means to be a dad and what it means to be masculine. Fathers are certainly special in their own way. But the two sexes are not the same.

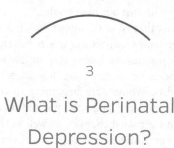

3

What is Perinatal Depression?

Understanding perinatal depression is not easy. Let me begin exploring this topic by busting some myths. Once we've worked out what it isn't, we can go on to look at what it is.

Eleven myths about PND

1. *It is caused by hormonal imbalance.* This theory stills holds very strong in our society. We are told that every woman should expect to feel sad and tearful about three days after the birth, while her hormones go through strong changes. This is a reflection of a long-held assumption in our society that women's hormones make us mad. Whether it be due to premenstrual syndrome, or mood swings during pregnancy, or problems caused by the menopause, women's hormones are regarded as problematic throughout our sexual cycle. In a society that believes that women's hormones always wreak havoc with their emotional state, it makes sense to presume that this inherent weakness of womanhood would be even stronger during the strongest manifestation of our femininity

– the time when we create a human being and sustain it singlehandedly with just our own bodies.

However, this theory is no longer holding water. As we begin to understand women's hormones better, we begin to see that our hormones are just as responsible for joy, peace, connection and love, as they are for anger, despair and emotional lability. Women are beginning to celebrate their hormonal cycle, and recognise the joy and love that can be associated with hormonal changes, as well as the frustration and tears that can sometimes accompany them. In the three days following birth, when there are many hormonal changes going on, do we have to presume that this is an unpleasant time? Could it not be the case that instead of 'baby blues', women experience 'baby schmooze'. As Emma described it, 'I remember my third day with my new baby quite vividly. I did indeed cry. I surprised myself because I was in a baby shop at the time and I didn't want others to see me crying. However, the thing that I remember about crying was that I was feeling so loved, so loving, so happy, so joyful, special and proud. We didn't have much money, and my husband had said to me that we should buy the beautiful gliding chair because I deserved it. I had made him proud, and he wanted to buy me something. I just burst into tears of gratitude, love, joy and pride. That was my "baby blues". My baby blues were simply lovely.'

2. *Depression is caused by a chemical imbalance in the brain.* This modern myth is still very strong. It has been put forward and strengthened by the pharmaceutical industry, which wants us to believe that the answer is in the form of drugs that correct the serotonin balance in the brain. However, it has always simply been a theory, and research has, as yet, been unable to demonstrate its validity. The brain's neurochemistry is simply

too complicated at present, and I suspect the answers are also too complicated to provide us with a simple 'disease model' to explain what causes depression. While the pharmaceutical industry spent money on research to demonstrate the effectiveness of antidepressants, this has not been replicated by independent studies, which find antidepressants to be as effective as placebo for low to moderate depression. There is a little more evidence to support the use of drugs for severe depression. Don't forget that the placebo effect is a very powerful healer – it is not 'imagined'. It really does generate tangible and measurable healing in the body. It is a great example of the mind-body connection in action.

3. *If you try hard enough, you can snap out of it.* This belief comes about, I think, from our misunderstanding about the difference between feeling low or fed up, and being depressed. We have all felt low and down and sorry for ourselves at times, but we have all had the experience of that feeling lifting when we talk to a friend, or get stuck into a job, or divert our thinking onto something more positive. However, with depression, these things don't lift the depression. To ask a depressed person to snap out of it, is like asking a person with a broken arm to 'just carry on playing tennis'. One of the things that I think is most damaging about this myth, is that it suggests that the depressed person is somehow choosing to stay depressed, and can make a choice to stop being depressed. If you have been depressed yourself, you will know that to think someone would choose this state is crazy. Being depressed is so horrible, that you would much rather have a broken arm!

4. *A depressed person is not stressed.* Research is beginning to show us that when people are in a depressed state, their body is in a state of constant stress. It may not seem like it,

because they are not outwardly jittery, or panicky, but their minds are preoccupied and their bodies are tense. This fits with an evolutionary model of depression, which views it as a state of 'shut down' in the face of danger or hopelessness. Babies exhibit this when they are left to cry it out. At some point, they stop. This is not necessarily a sign that they are okay. They may have gone into a depressed state of shutting down, in the face of having no other options, while still feeling stressed or unsafe. Therapists are now realising that the first job of therapy, when working with a depressed person, is to help them to learn to relax. This will impact on their mood, their hormones, and lead to more restorative sleep patterns.

5. *It only affects women.* This is not true. In some studies, rates of perinatal depression in fathers have been found to be as high as those for mothers. Men are suffering too. And the rates that they are suffering, seem to be dramatically on the increase. Reasons for why this might be so are outlined in Chapter 4, but most of the book applies to you if you are a soon-to-be father.

6. *It is not as serious as physical problems.* Depression is a major problem in our society, and continues to grow. Estimates are that 1 in 3 women and 1 in 5 men will suffer from depression in their lifetime. Postnatal depression is said to affect between 10 and 50 per cent of women, and between 10 and 15 per cent of men. It is the leading cause of death in women in the perinatal period. Yes, you read that right. You are more likely to die from suicide perinatally, than from any other childbirth-related complication. That, in my book, makes it pretty serious.

7. *There's no cure.* The problem with depression is that people often feel stuck with it, believing that it is a part of their

personality, and not treatable. However, psychology and medicine have made great progress in finding ways to relieve, if not treat altogether, symptoms of depression. Furthermore, perinatal depression often lifts spontaneously – given that it is, to some extent, a reaction to difficult life circumstances. When the difficult life circumstances get easier, and when we begin to adjust to change, our mood lifts accordingly. Thus, perinatal depression does get better, and it gets better quicker with help from others, be that family, a GP, or a therapist.

8. *It stops you loving your baby.* I've often heard women tell me that they knew something was wrong, but they didn't think it could be postnatal depression, because 'I loved my baby so much'. You can have depression and still love your baby very much. It is common for depression to 'numb' loving feelings, but it is not necessarily so.

9. *It doesn't affect normal, healthy, successful people.* Some people think that a mental illness affects people who were already faltering in some way, whereas something like cancer can strike anyone. Thus, they are more afraid of cancer. This is evidenced in the funding and resources that go into cancer research when compared with mental health research. While I know that cancer needs money for research, I do wish that as much money was raised for researching depression as it is for researching cancer. In the US, the National Institutes of Health pumped about 5.3 billion dollars into cancer research in 2013, and only 2.2 billion into mental health research as a whole (with only 415 million of that going towards depression). In the UK, the European Union invested about 54.3 million Euros for studies of mental health disorders, and 205 million for studies of cancer. The reasons are not to do with which disorder is more devastating for personal lives or the economy. It has to

do with stigma, and, I believe, the erroneous assumption that cancer can strike for *anybody*, including people 'like me', but mental health problems only strike 'other people'. So the fear of getting cancer is stronger in us, and motivates us to put funding forward to prevent and treat it. However, it simply isn't true. Depression and mental health problems affect up to 50 per cent of mothers at any one time. And up to 30 per cent of us over a lifetime. And it kills people too. It strikes and can kill normal healthy successful intelligent people like you and me.

10. *If you have postnatal depression, you are somehow weaker than others.* The people I have met who have perinatal depression are strong. The condition can be so debilitating, that even getting out of bed takes an enormous amount of determination and strength, let alone getting through the rest of the day. Mothers who carry on parenting when they feel so disabled by an awful horrific feeling that they can't explain to others, or help others understand, are, in my book, pretty awesomely amazing. And as you will come to see from this book, a lot of perinatal depression is about lack of support and lack of celebration and respect, for the incredibly demanding job that is mothering a new baby in a society that has lost its 'village'. Women and men who are depressed are having to be an awful lot stronger than those who aren't, just to get through the day.

11. *If you suffer postnatal depression, you will damage your baby.* This belief is about as helpful as the belief that if you are stressed during your pregnancy you are damaging your baby. It is far too generalised, far too black and white, and very unhelpful. The very fact that society loves to peddle this scientific generalisation is an example to me of how much guilt and responsibility we put on the shoulders of already stressed mothers. It is true that there is a vague statistical

pattern that exists, but this doesn't tell us anything about you and your baby. For example, there's a pattern that exists to show us that having pets in the home helps reduce asthma. I don't have pets in my home, so can I blame that on why my child has asthma? Absolutely not, because asthma is far more complicated than that in real life. With postnatal depression, I can't tell you how many women tell me that their baby or child grew into a happy, delightful, interactive, intelligent little gem.

What is perinatal depression?

This might sound crazy, but we don't actually know what perinatal depression is! There. I've admitted it. Many professionals will be cross with me, shouting at the book that 'We DO know what it is, we know what causes it, we know how to treat it!' I agree that there are many experts out there who spend their whole lives studying depression, listening deeply and intimately to people who are depressed, studying the hormonal, endocrine, neurological, immunological systems, analysing sleep patterns of depressed people, theorising about the evolutionary mechanisms of depression, and others who are treating people who are depressed with great success. They save many lives. However, I maintain that there is very little agreement on what it actually *is*. I guess the reason for this, as outlined in the introduction, is because depression is multi-faceted: it is a product of our culture (making it difficult for us to 'see'), and it is not psychological *or* physical, but both. Experts can't even agree on whether perinatal depression is the same, or completely different to, non-perinatal depression.

Although we don't really know what perinatal depression is, the work that the 'experts' are doing is not in vain. We have managed to come a long way in understanding it, recognising it, and making it better. We will now take a look at what seems to cause depression, how you can recognise it in yourself and others, how you can prevent it, and what you can do if you are suffering from it.

Let's begin with what it feels like.

What depression feels like

If you ask a psychiatrist how to diagnose depression, he or she will tell you the following (according to the *Diagnostic and Statistical Manual of Mental Disorders*, the most popular reference guide for psychiatrists and psychologists in the UK):

Firstly, the person either needs to feel low, OR they need to find no enjoyment in things any more.

Feeling low is the main marker of depression. For a diagnosis, this feeling needs to be ongoing for at least two weeks. It is not always the case that someone who is depressed will say that they feel low.

Being unable to enjoy things is known as *anhedonia*. You don't enjoy doing things any more, and you don't look forward to doing things any more either. The joy has gone. Sometimes, this is the feeling that people are most aware of, more than feeling low. In this case, they might not really be aware that they are depressed.

Just one of the above has to be present, in order to meet the criteria for diagnosis. There is a difference between *lacking* a positive feeling (when there's an absence of joy, or a sense of emptiness) and a negative feeling being *present* (such as being very down or irritable). You can have one, or both, when you are depressed.

Then there are many other 'symptoms' that are common with depression, which include the following:

- Change in appetite – eating less, or eating more, leading to significant weight change

- Changes in sleep patterns – either not being able to sleep, or sleeping a lot and still feeling like it isn't enough
- Changes in activity – restless and agitated or slowed down
- Tiredness and loss of energy
- Feelings of worthlessness or excessive or inappropriate guilt
- Problems concentrating, 'fuzzy' head, or difficulty making decisions
- Thoughts of death or suicide
- Anxiety symptoms such as irrational worry, trouble relaxing, feeling tense

The above symptoms will differ according to your specific experiences of depression. Some people will notice feelings of guilt or self-loathing more than others, or you might be mostly aware of feeling drained of all energy. What does seem to be the case for everyone, and isn't really obvious in the psychiatrists' manuals, is the *struggle* to get through the day. Each day feels like an enormous, 'wading through treacle' effort, both physically and emotionally. As Christine put it, 'Day to day life with PND feels like a never-ending walk through a thick heavy swamp, disinteresting, monotonous and the hardest walk of your life'.

Many people who have experienced depression liken it to a dark cloud having descended over you. In this way, depression feels like a very physical thing that happens 'to you', much like a sore throat happens 'to you'. As Karla put it, 'Everything always felt so dark, almost like all I can remember is darkness all the time, like I was living with no light'.

Another hallmark of depression is the sense of being stuck, and that things will never change (what we professionals call 'hopelessness'). That is one of the many reasons that feeling suicidal is a common symptom of depression, because the only way you can think of to escape the awful feelings is to not exist anymore. As Emma put it, 'Your life plays in slow motion and every minute feels like hours. Like your life is literally coming to an end and the worst part of it is that you can't wait for it to happen'. The feeling of hopelessness is strong in depression, and is a strong causal factor in feeling suicidal. But *it is not true* that you are stuck and hopeless. Depression is an illness, just like any other, and depression gets better, just like any other illness. When you are better, your life will feel very different, and you will be able to enjoy things with energy once more, and feel that you deserve to do so. Remember that HOPE stands for 'Hold On, Pain Ends'.

A feeling of loneliness is also common with depression. The loneliness is not actually about how alone you are, it is about how alone you *feel*, so you can feel very lonely even when you are surrounded by people. As Lauri put it, 'I felt lonely, even when I was surrounded by wonderful supportive family and friends'. Loneliness is often accompanied by a sense that no one understands. 'I feel so alone because your friends and family have no idea how to understand what you're going through'.

Added factors for perinatal and postnatal depression

There is no recognised difference between depression which you might get after your baby is born (postnatal depression), depression which you might get during your pregnancy and up to four weeks after your baby is born (perinatal depression) and depression which you might get at any other point in your life.

In other words, we don't really understand whether they are all the same thing, or whether there is something distinct or different about perinatal depression. There are a few other feelings or 'symptoms' which are particularly prevalent when depression strikes around the time that a baby is born. These include overwhelming responsibility, guilt, bonding problems, grief and loss.

Overwhelming responsibility

Feeling overwhelmed with responsibility is very common with perinatal depression because there is an obvious target for it – the wellbeing of your little one. Parenting is a very difficult job, and is impossible to get right. Despite this, our society puts an awful lot of pressure on us to be 'perfect parents', by making us aware of the many ways that we can 'damage' our babies. News reports seem to be riddled with ways in which children can be harmed by their mothers, and it begins in pregnancy. You can eat the wrong things, smell the wrong things, be too stressed, be too heavy, weigh too little, be too sad, drink the wrong things... Then, when the baby is born, we are given conflicting advice about dummies, sleep positions, foods, when to wean, baby routines, slings, temperature of rooms, mattresses, drinking cups, medicines and so on. It really is a minefield of potential worry and confusion. In the past, a mother might have looked to her nearest and dearest for advice and expertise. After all, her own parents had done it all before, and they genuinely care about the baby too. Her family could show her how it is done, show her how resilient babies actually are, show her how not to be too anxious or scared. However, in our modern culture, the burden of responsibility lies with the mother and father, not with grandparents or aunties or older sisters. Also, the 'expert' advice has changed so quickly and so dramatically over the years that the grandparents' opinion is no longer valued. For example, psychologists introduced the notion that babies should have strict feeding schedules (in line with the behaviourists' principles of conditioning) in the 1960s. There has now been a complete U-turn on this, with experts now saying that babies need to be fed on demand, and must not be left to cry. My mother has never heard that I can 'damage' my baby by leaving him to cry, and so she, and her advice, has become effectively muted. In our modern society, we have lost the support and reassurance that previous generations would have got from their families. Mothers' wisdom has been stolen by the experts and the professionals. So we can no longer turn to the woman who cares about you the most, who has done it before herself, and who genuinely cares about your baby more than any other expert. New parents no longer have the rich source of reassurance and support that they might have had in previous generations. And so they have an awful lot of responsibility on their shoulders! Tracey told me of her 'constant fear that you'll damage your child and you have no idea what you are doing'. This enormous sense of responsibility in the face of not really knowing how to do the job of looking after your baby (because you've never done it before) leads to feeling overwhelmed, or a feeling of 'drowning'. As Sarah put it 'I thought Will was going to die so I didn't sleep for weeks in case he stopped breathing'. This struggle to cope, and feeling overwhelmed, often links directly to a sense of guilt.

Guilt and worthlessness

Feeling worthless and guilty is common in depression, but I think new mothers and fathers are particularly vulnerable to it, because having a new baby leaves you feeling confused, tired, inept, chaotic, constantly chasing your tail and never being able to finish anything. Thus, the demands of looking after a new baby, looking after yourself, learning on the job, not getting a moment's rest, looking after a house and being frightened of getting any little thing wrong, creates an awful lot of room for guilt! We all naturally want to do the best for our baby. It is built into our evolutionary wiring. We all become anxious if we think that we are not doing the best for our baby. It is natural. On top of this, you might already be a bit of a perfectionist, or quite hard on yourself. This can add to the pressure you are under, and your sense of guilt. Sarah says, 'I felt so worthless and such a bad mother for not coping'. I have even heard women talk of feeling guilty because they don't feel guilty! If you feel guilty (and I've not often met a mother who doesn't feel guilt), please remember that this does not mean that you are bad, or worthless, or not good enough. *Feeling* guilty and *being* guilty are two very different things! When the depression lifts, mothers can often see that it was the depression making them feel guilty, and that they were actually perfectly good enough as a mother. As Stacey put it 'I felt as though I was a terrible mother for not being able to breastfeed. I felt worthless and just wanted to disappear, then I felt even worse because I was sure my moods were affecting everyone else. I can see now that I really shouldn't have beaten myself up over not being able to breastfeed as my children are healthy and happy'. Depression makes you *feel* guilty, it does not mean that you *are* guilty.

Bonding issues with your baby

Depression eats up good feelings. Feelings of love and joy are replaced with feelings of emptiness or sadness or anger and anxiety. This means that it can be difficult to feel loving and affectionate towards anyone, including your new baby. Furthermore, nature has programmed us to feel a particular kind of protectiveness and love towards our own babies, and this happens most strongly around the time of birth. If this 'programming' was missed due to a difficult birth, or the presence of depression, then it may be even harder to bond with your baby. As Danielle put it 'I didn't want my little girl any more and resented doing anything for her'. Rest assured that it is the depression that is interrupting your ability to feel love for your baby, and that when the depression lifts, the feelings will resurface, or you will fall in love with your baby for the first time.

Overwhelmed by anxiety for your baby's welfare

Some people think that they can't be depressed because they feel a fierce, deep and protective love for their baby. It may be that your depression has not affected your ability to bond with your baby at all. On the contrary, it is your strong bond with your baby that is exacerbating the many negative feelings of anxiety, guilt, panic and despair. You may be frantic about your baby's wellbeing, and struggle to let anyone else hold her, or feel that you can't go out of the house with her because the outside world is too dangerous for you both. This makes it very difficult for you to relax, leading to exhaustion and depression.

A difficult birth

Becoming a new mother often begins when a difficult birth ends. I am a birth doula, and after a night of attending a birth, I go home and recover. It can take quite a while! I always wonder how in heaven's name the mother is ever going to recover, because I feel battered and I don't have a baby to look after! If, on top of tiredness, you have negative feelings about the birth, such as disappointment, horror or shock, then recovery is even harder. Some women and men are left with strong traumatic symptoms after the birth, and need time to process and heal psychologically. You are not alone if you feel like this. However, it is also very common to come away from your birth feeling delighted, proud, loved-up and awesome, so please don't feel discouraged if you are awaiting your baby's birth. Nature designed us to give birth awash with a cocktail of 'ecstatic birth hormones' (Sarah Buckley), and you are no different.

Grief and loss

When we become parents, our role changes, and our life changes. There are things that we cannot get back, such as our old carefree, independent, organised lives. For some people, the sense of loss is such that they feel that they have actually lost a part of who they are, and that it has been subsumed into the role of 'mother'. As Vick puts it, 'I would do anything to go back to life before I had the baby. Like I'm in mourning for what my life was like before I had her'. Helen talks about the loss of identity: 'I had no idea who I was any more, I totally lost my identity. I was just a mum, and I was being dictated to totally by this tiny person'. Grief and loss have long been known to be associated with depression. This problem is partly caused by our culture, because there is so much negativity around about having babies. Young people are often warned that when they become parents they will 'throw their lives away'. Feminists warned us in the 1970s that motherhood is a boring, thankless task that strips you of your identity. I would even go so far as to say that motherhood is regarded as fairly worthless and low-status in our society. And yet, it is arguably the most difficult and the most important job in the world. Imagine if our society *really* believed this? Imagine if society gave new parents due awe and respect, and helped them to make parenting easier.

Mums would get the best seats on the planes, not be stuck in the back having to cope with people rolling their eyes at them. There would be special seats on trains for mums too, with all that they need to make their job easier. It would be much easier to get a job if 'mother' was on your CV, because people would immediately credit you with patience, flexibility, maturity, selflessness, organisational skills and more. You would be granted time to do this important job, and be treated with respect and deference while you were doing it. As soon as you became a new parent, your self-esteem would increase, you would feel special and amazing, and you would say good riddance to the 'old' you that was just 'a nobody'. You would know that you were special, because people would look up to you, admire you, meet your needs. As a new mother, you would presume that you are far too important to hoover or mop toilets. You, and only you, are needed by your baby to bring up a functional and healthy baby for humanity's good. Cleaning toilets can be done by others. It's fanciful thinking, but if a CEO can think like that, why can't a woman with the most important and difficult job in the world think like that?

The impending birth

Fear of birth is a growing phenomenon in our culture, and there is even a name for severe fear – tokophobia. It can make for a very scary and unhappy pregnancy. It comes in many forms, but the one that is most associated with depression is known as antenatal tokophobia. You might have really wanted a baby, and been delighted to become pregnant, only to find yourself feeling deep dread and misery whenever you think about the birth. As Stacey put it: 'I was planning for a baby and I really wanted one, so when I was so upset from the moment I found out I was pregnant my feelings really scared me. I cried for about 36 hours without stopping. I completely withdrew from most people as I couldn't handle people being excited about my baby when I wasn't. I felt I was abnormal. I felt so scared for myself and upset, I would cry every day.' Stacey sought emotional support from professionals to help deal with her fear of the birth, and this helped a lot. She went on to enjoy her birth and early motherhood. It is very common to be depressed antenatally and for this to lift after you have had the baby, so if you are pregnant and miserable it does not necessarily mean that you will suffer from depression after your baby is born.

Your changing body

Many women love the feeling of being pregnant, and the changes that come with it. Many women feel alive, gorgeous and proud. However, if this isn't you, don't worry: you are not alone. You might feel sad for the loss of your previous slim figure, or worried about permanent changes that may or may not happen, or simply very uncomfortable and unhappy with being pregnant. Feelings about your body may contribute to depression if you are freaked out by your growing baby, or horrified by the changes taking place. Your body is not your own any more, and people may feel compelled to touch your bump without asking, which can feel like an invasion of privacy. Note that this is an evolutionary instinct. When someone touches your bump, they are welcoming your baby, connecting with your baby and celebrating your baby. It is a tribal instinct that stays very strong in us, but in our modern, private lives, it can cause offence. Try not to be offended. You could try to see it as a loving and welcoming gesture, albeit clumsily carried out.

Fear of the unknown, and no going back

I don't even like putting a letter in a post-box, because once it's done, I can't get it back. Being pregnant can lead to feelings of being trapped with no way out, because you cannot slow, halt, or rush the growth of your bump, or the time that the baby will take to be born. This lack of control may be new for you, and may lead to feelings of anxiety or helplessness. If this is the case for you, find ways to help yourself, such as going to positive birth groups, or talking to people that help you to feel more optimistic and excited about your journey.

Feeling vulnerable and confused

When we become pregnant, we get 'booked in' to the NHS, bloods are taken, we are asked which hospital we will go to, we are given more hospital appointments for 'checks' and we are advised on things we can and can't eat. Meanwhile, the rest of the world imparts their advice, most of which is contradictory. And to boot, people will share their horror birth stories, or crack jokes like 'Get lots of sleep now because you won't know what's hit you when that baby comes'. And that is just real life. We then have the internet to add salt to the wound. At a time when the world should be celebrating with you, making you feel special and sharing in your excitement, we are testing you and scaring you. This adds to feelings of vulnerability and confusion, increasing your chances of feeling low, tearful and depressed.

Fathers feeling rushed

For the mother, her body's changes are a constant reminder of the impending arrival of the baby. However, fathers are in a peculiar situation because they do not have these bodily changes. Pregnancy can be especially surreal for them, and they may find it difficult to appreciate that a real life baby is on the way. It can take fathers a little longer to adjust mentally to the fact that they are going to be a parent. This can create feelings of pressure or loss of control, as they may feel guilty for not making attempts to bond with the baby, or not going to antenatal classes, or not being as excited as quickly as the mother. Fathers need time to adjust to the immense changes that will be coming their way, and they also need time to adjust to the transformation of their partner's body. This can be difficult while they are still holding down a full-time job, trying to support their partner and preparing the house. Conversely, if they are really excited and keen to get involved, they might find that the NHS isn't quite as open and receptive as they had hoped, and they end up feeling like a spare part at the antenatal meetings.

On the whole, having depression feels awful. The worst thing about it, is that no one else can see it or relate to it. If you are in an accident, and have a swollen black eye and a broken arm to show for it, people will fuss over you, do things for you, and sympathise. If you are told by the doctor that you have pneumonia, people will fuss over you, do things for you and sympathise. They can't see pneumonia, but somehow they can relate to it. It is an illness which takes time to heal. But if we have been told that we have depression, the reaction is sometimes very different. People can't see it, they don't understand it and they can't relate to it.

Birth trauma and post-traumatic stress disorder

Up to 60 per cent of women report a 'negative birth experience', with up to 25 per cent saying they felt traumatised by their births. Experts put the rate of full-blown post-traumatic stress disorder (PTSD) at about 2 to 5 per cent for men and women. When trauma presents, the person feels as if it has just happened, and the body and brain are in a state of hyper-arousal. This might involve nightmares, flashbacks, irritability, moodiness, tearfulness, sleep problems, anger with your loved ones, constant memories of the incident and unsuccessful efforts to push it out of your mind. If you are a new parent, there are even more consequences, because it can interrupt the process of bonding with your baby. Furthermore, the normal chaos that comes with adjusting to a new baby is heightened to create a potentially miserable cocktail. Fathers can be traumatised by the birth too, but this often goes under the radar. After a difficult birth, mothers and fathers need time and tender loving care to help the mind process the event. This can take weeks or months. When the brain 'gets stuck' and doesn't seem to be healing from the nightmares or flashbacks or anxiety, it might be PTSD.

If you think you have been traumatised by your baby's birth, then please know that it is very treatable. Treatment options and some self-help techniques are covered in Chapter 5.

What causes depression?

Experts can't agree on what depression is. Neither can they agree on what causes depression. There are many theories out there, but for the time being I think it helps to think of it like this:

Something in you is not right. Things are out of balance, and you need to think about how to get back in balance. This is not just a physical thing. It is not just a psychological thing. It is not just a cultural thing. It is all three, because all these three are interconnected. Changing one aspect will affect the others, though this might take time.

Physically, you might focus on your sleep, or your diet, or on exercise. Psychologically, you might practise mindfulness, or self-compassion, or relaxation, or affirmations, or become more assertive, or work on your sense of inferiority. Socially, you might join a club and get out more, or make a decision to stop seeing people who get you down, or make an effort to see people who help you feel better.

Some interesting theories about what causes depression

There is a lot of work going on at the moment to work out what causes depression. Unlike malaria, which has only one cause, depression throws us a curve ball because it seems to have numerous causes. As with cancer, we don't know what exactly is causing the problem, but we have some really good evidence pointing to some specific triggers or risk factors. Here are some potential causes of depression:

Depression is caused by your earliest interactions

The way you were looked after as a baby and toddler seems to be related to the risk of developing depression. We know that if you were neglected or emotionally abused, it can upset the wiring of your brain and nervous system. This impacts on our ability to relate to others in a trusting, relaxed, mutually beneficial way. For example, research has shown us that oxytocin (the loving, connecting, bonding hormone) acts differently in people who have had abusive childhoods. Loving connection does not soothe them; it activates their threat system, because their brain has learned that the people who are supposed to love you end up hurting you.

When you've had a rough babyhood, the brain seems to become hard wired for stress, and responds very quickly and very easily with stress hormones, even in situations which would not stress others. The stress response can be one of 'freeze', whereby your brain and nervous system simply give up and dissolve into a state of hopelessness and despair. This is not something that you can control, any more than you can control your eyelids closing when you sneeze.

Learning that the way we were treated as children might have made us more vulnerable to anxiety and depression might sound fatalistic and upsetting. However, I would like you to see it a different way. The main thing to take from it is to know that *it is not your fault*. You did not choose your life. You did not even choose to be born. From the moment that you were born, you were surviving as best you could. And you continue to do that. Now that you are an adult, you have much more control than you did as a baby, and you can choose to turn your life around, slowly but surely.

Depression is caused by social inequality and poverty

The clearest causal factor that increases your chances of developing depression is inequality and poverty. We know that people below the poverty line in the USA have twice as much incidence of depression as those not below the poverty line. However, it would seem that the significant factor isn't how poor you are *per se*, it is how poor you are *relative* to those around you. Relatively high levels of depression among the poor are found in those countries that have the worst inequality (gulf between rich and poor). These countries have the highest overall rates of mental illness, and it is increased among the poor (research by Richard Wilkinson). It is not just about how much money or food you have, it is about status and social position. You may not think this factor is relevant to you because you are actually doing okay in the wealth and social status stakes, but I beg to differ. It does affect you, because this is a universal psychological phenomenon at play – that of *status insecurity*.

Depression is a symptom of status insecurity

Have you ever noticed yourself comparing yourself to others?

And have you noticed that when you do so, you almost always feel worse? Have you noticed that on a 'bad day', you are more likely to do it? Social comparison, or mentally comparing yourself to others, is a normal part of our psychology. Because it is normal and automatic, we can let it run away with us, and it can contribute to feelings of inadequacy, low mood, and cut across our feelings of warmth towards people.

Paul Gilbert outlined many years ago a theory of depression that puts social rank, or social status, in the spotlight. He argues that depression is a reaction to feeling 'down-graded' socially, or to having lost respect, value or esteem in the eyes of others (whether or not the sufferer has *actually* been down-ranked is irrelevant, it is how the person *feels*). This really matters to humans, because being liked, accepted and valued by others is the evolutionary key to our survival and success. It is built into our psychological wiring. We are social beings, and we survive and thrive on mutual connection, support, touch, play and interaction. No man is an island. However, if our friends turn against us, we are better off on an island, because humans can do an awful lot of harm to our psychological and emotional wellbeing.

The effects of being bullied can be devastating to our emotional wellbeing. Being singled out by a large group is potentially even more devastating. This is a throwback to when we lived in much smaller hunter-gatherer groups. If the group turned against us, it threatened our very survival. Even though we now live in much bigger groups, and it is easier to avoid people who don't value us, we still have an inbuilt desire to be liked, wanted, valued, respected and sought after. How you seek that respect depends upon the type of person that you are. You might want to be seen to look great, to have a nice house, to be doing an interesting job, to be a good parent, to be invited to parties, to be asked to look after someone's dog, to be described as caring, or clever and so on. This inbuilt need to be accepted, valued and respected is not a problem while all is well, and it drives us to improve ourselves and get on with those around us. But it can turn toxic. The part of our psychology that is concerned with social status can go into overdrive. Status insecurity can lead us to believe that we are not worthy of respect, that others are better than us, that no matter what we do, we can never be good enough. We can start to believe that we are not lovable or worthy of love. We can begin to feel that other people are better, more successful or happier than us. We can feel angry, cheated and let down because life is throwing us a raw deal.

If you haven't already noticed, this is a hallmark of depression – feeling worthless and hopeless. Gilbert calls this our 'tricky brains' in action. He argues that depression is an involuntary evolutionary mechanism, whereby you stop trying to be better than others (express hopelessness or suicidality), by 'accepting' or 'believing' that you are worthless, and thereby submitting to others. This protects you from being killed or cast out by your group. As with a lot of evolved mechanisms, such as the fight or flight reaction, our environment has changed faster than our biology, and so we are victims of a psychological system that we no longer need, but can't switch off. Our 'tricky brains' give us more than we bargained for.

Here is the link between social inequality and status insecurity: in societies where there is a bigger gap between rich and poor, there seems to be more status insecurity, leading to more mental illness. In the case of parenting, I would argue that being a single mother is held in very low social status by our society. We know that being a single mother increases your risk of depression. But we can't be sure why. Richard Wilkinson's work on inequality suggests that it is not the poverty *per se* that is a risk factor, but the low social status that comes with being a single mother. I would take that a step further, and say that parenting as a whole has low value in our society. As such, parents are much more likely to compare themselves with others, to question and doubt themselves, to express resentment and anger towards other parents, and to feel inadequate, trapped and depressed. The answers lie at many levels. Societally, we need to be more equal. Within our closer communities, we need to celebrate and value motherhood and fatherhood. Within your own psychology, we can do some personal work on getting to know our 'tricky brains'. This involves recognising the difference between 'I feel inadequate' and 'I am inadequate'. They are not the same. Acceptance is also important. Do not blame yourself for your tricky thinking, just like you wouldn't blame yourself for getting a bruise.

Survive not thrive system

As mentioned in the section about babies bonding, we can either be in a 'survive' or 'thrive' state of mind. The survival system is nature's way of protecting us, by switching on our 'threat' or 'alarm' system. This is associated with the hormones adrenalin and cortisol, and with emotions of fear, panic, anger, jealousy, and depression. None of these feel good, but they didn't evolve to feel good. They evolved to feel bad, so that you would do something to protect yourself (even if that involved laying low, hiding and doing nothing). The 'thrive' system is divided up into two areas, one of which is the soothing, or calming system. This is associated with relaxed, loving, calm, chilled-out, dozy, 'lie back in the sun and do nothing' feelings. These *do* feel good, and we are motivated to relax, sleep and take it easy as much as possible, but *only if it is safe to do so*! Meerkats don't sleep if there's a tiger about. Neither do humans. If we suddenly remember that we didn't finish our assignment, our relaxation is broken.

With depression, the theory is that our relaxation is constantly broken, and we can't settle, rest or enjoy that 'lie back in the sun and do nothing' feeling. What stops us doing things isn't a feeling of relaxation, it is a feeling of paralysis, tension and doubt, like a rabbit stuck in the headlights. With depression, the strategy seems to be keeping yourself out of the spotlight, laying low, not taking any risks, not challenging anyone, believing that you are inadequate to avoid confrontation and so on. These are hallmarks of the depressive threat system in action. You did not do anything to switch this system on. You cannot control it. It is not your fault. It is a normal, automatic, human reaction to perceived threat.

All sorts of things can switch on the depressive threat system: fear of failing, money worries, boredom, lack of sleep, too much to do, people being unkind to us. So with depression, our 'alarm' system is constantly switched on. This literally stops the good feelings getting in, because nature prioritises survival over feeling good. The good feelings that are stopped include loving feelings (Is the world safe enough to trust people?), fun and joy (Can I really focus on playing, when I'm not even sure I have any dinner for my family?), relaxation (If I close my eyes, I'm vulnerable to attack).

It's really important to understand that the human mind isn't reacting to Stone Age threats of 'tigers in the bushes' any more. But it is reacting strongly to threats to our social connections and social status. This is so pervasive, and so human, that we are not even aware of it most of the time. Start paying attention to this possibility, and you will notice it more and more. Worrying about doing that talk, unsure about what your boss makes of you, wanting to wear the appropriate clothes for the party, wanting to be seen to be talented, mulling over whether you said the right thing or not yesterday, wanting people to think you are a great mum, not sure whether you took the right job or not, trying to work out why someone said something to you, and what they meant, feeling that you're missing out on life when you go on Facebook, being annoyed because someone didn't respond to your text, and so on.

Please remember that none of this is our fault. It is how we are wired evolutionarily, historically and circumstantially. Evolutionarily, we are biased to spot the negatives and be alert to danger. Historically, you might have been dealt a raw deal in terms of your babyhood or toddlerhood, affecting the ease with which your nervous system clicks into 'threat' mode. Circumstantially, you are in a society which doesn't value motherhood, and you may be dealing with other stressors such as poverty, loneliness, or unkind friends and family. None of this is your fault. It is nature's automatic protection system. You did not ask it to be switched on, and you cannot control the on switch. It just happened, like a runny nose happens when we get a cold.

It is not your fault, but what can you do about it? There are many established ways of helping you to switch off your survival system and bring yourself into the joy/relaxation system. They are exercises for the mind, and they take time and practice, just like exercises for the body take time and practice before you notice the effect. Also, once you start to notice the benefits, you need to keep at it, or your body and mind will revert to the default position. (There is more about this in Chapter 5, Everyday Psychological Wellbeing Techniques.)

Depression as a symptom of unmet emotional needs

Joe Griffin and Ivan Tyrrell put forward a compelling argument that almost all cases of depression boil down to unmet emotional needs. As humans, we have physical needs such as warmth, food and water. However, we also have emotional needs, and when these aren't met, we get poorly. The Human Givens approach outlines nine basic emotional needs. As you read through these, have a think about which of them might be most pertinent to you:

1. *The need for security.* According to the Human Givens approach, financial security, such as being free of money worries, is as important as personal security, such as being free of abuse or bullying. Both can impact on depression. When we have a baby, our need for security can be heightened. Financially, we are likely to have money worries. We might have to take time off work, or buy things for the baby, or get a decent roof over our heads. We need to think about the future, taking on financial responsibility for another human being and so on. Emotionally, we are likely to feel scared that the baby is not safe in our hands. This, as outlined above, is because we are left alone as a couple with the baby a lot, and also, there is a great deal of information out there in magazines and on the internet about possible dangers to your baby. That does not help us feel more secure! I remember one couple I worked with had bought three different thermometers because they were so worried about the room temperature being perfect for the baby, due to things they had read in magazines. It didn't occur to them that babies in Africa and Iceland fare just fine, despite there being no thermometers in their rooms. We know that women who are in abusive relationships are more likely to experience depression. Their need for security is not being met.

2. *The need for attention.* The second emotional need, according to the Human Givens model, is that of attention. In our society we tend to denigrate the need for attention, but

it is so important to our healthy psychological functioning to feel that we get enough good quality attention from others, and to be able to give it too. You might think that you will get a lot more attention when you have a baby, and that might well be true. If it is true, enjoy it, because you really do deserve it. However, it might be that your baby is getting all the attention, and you are expected to take second place. For example, many women feel that they aren't given the chance to really talk about their birth (which is a very special event in any woman's life) because 'the baby is here now and that is all that matters'. Or maybe you simply feel that people don't really notice you any more. I remember one new mum telling me that people never looked at her because they were so busy looking at the baby. Furthermore, I think the drop in attention is even stronger for fathers. Not only are they playing second fiddle to the baby, but they are also playing second fiddle to the mother. Plus, they have lost the mother's attention, as well as that of well-meaning visitors and professionals. As I said earlier, the need for attention isn't well understood in our society, and we tend to think badly of people who need it. But this is to misunderstand that, young or old, we all need good-quality attention from the people around us. You, and your partner, need good-quality attention from each other, from your family, from your friends, and from professionals. Do not underestimate or play down your need for this.

3. *The need for control.* In order to be free of depression, we all need to have some control over our lives and the decisions we can and cannot make. To not be able to do this is known to be very toxic and stressful. We can lose control of our finances by going into debt, or of our bodies if we are suffering panic attacks, or of everyday things if we live

with a controlling partner. The need for control is always challenged when a baby enters the picture. This is because you lose control over normal everyday routines such as when to eat, when to sleep, when to shower and when to go to the toilet. This sudden loss of control can be more difficult if you were used to having a lot of control previously – for example, if you were quite an independent or autonomous person beforehand. If you feel this will be a challenge for you, or you are currently struggling with this, just be aware that you are not unusual. This is a difficult adaptation, and it will get easier.

4. *The need for emotional connectedness.* Having one or more people in our lives that we feel very close to fulfils a basic need to be connected to others in an intimate way. We can relax with people without worrying about how we are coming across, and this helps us feel safe, nurtured and content. Hopefully, this will become stronger for you when you have a baby. A lot of couples feel that they connect more strongly to their partner, and grow closer as they share this adventure. You may also find that you grow closer to your own parents, given that you are going through the same adventure that they did, so many years ago. And of course, your love for your baby also creates an emotional connection that you didn't even have before! However, if this is not the case for you, then it might be because feelings of depression can thwart loving feelings. In this case, it is the depression that is the problem – not you. Once the depression lifts, your loving feelings will come back.

5. *The need for community.* According to the Human Givens model, the need to feel part of something bigger than our immediate family goes back to our ancestral roots. This

helps us feel that we belong, that our lives are meaningful, and that we are safe. Without this basic need being met, we can struggle. Your sense of belonging to and being part of a group can be enhanced when you have a baby. You can feel proud of being a parent, and excited by the stories and experiences of others, looking forward to joining baby groups and meeting other parents. Many new parents will tell you that spending time with others in the same situation as you (in other words, joining the community) is a very important part of coping with a new baby. Being able to socialise with others who understand and can support you, appears to be incredibly valuable to new parents. Isolation is not helpful. Although it can be difficult to get out of the house on a regular basis (especially if you are depressed) it can be something that really helps lift mood and helps you feel that you do belong somewhere and you are not alone. Community is important, and when you have a baby, you have an opportunity to become part of a new one.

6. *The need for privacy.* Every now and again, we need peace, quiet and privacy in order to give the brain space to literally process what is going on. Things that happen to us on the outside need to be processed and made sense of on the inside. For this, we need moments of peace, quiet and privacy. Your need for privacy can be much harder to meet when you have a baby. A lot of new mums know what it feels like to crave time to be alone. Having ten minutes to shower is often impossible, and the dream of sitting for five minutes to enjoy a cup of tea is often history. Please don't be frightened by this. Neither should you think it won't affect you. The point is that these needs are just that. Needs. We might think we can go without water while we climb Everest, but the reality is that we will start to feel the need for water

very acutely. Similarly, we might think that we can have a baby and not need privacy, but at some point you will start to pine for it. Being aware of this (rather than frightened by it) means that you can build ways to meet all of these needs into your life when you have a baby. If you already have a baby, you can think about whether this need is strong for you, or whether it is being met for you. If not, that might be one reason why you are struggling.

7. *The need to maintain status.* This concerns the need to feel important, valued, respected and generally okay in the eyes of others. If there has been a dramatic change in this, and you feel you have lost status, this can be emotionally damaging and lead to depression. When we have a baby, it helps if we can feel proud, valued, cherished, and important. I remember a friend saying to me once 'I feel so proud of myself, like I've done something absolutely amazing, even though women do it all the time'.

Many societies celebrate this time in a couple's life, and help the couple feel good about themselves and their contribution to society. However, in our society it is a double-edged sword. How we actually treat women does not give them the message that they are especially valuable or special. We rob them of their privacy and dignity during the birth process, then leave them on a ward full of other crying babies, take their husbands from them for the night, leave them with minimal help due to busy staff and then send them home, regardless of whether they have support at home or not. Many women are frightened of even becoming mothers, due to fear of the birth, and fear of the stresses of parenthood in terms of what it does to our bodies and our identities. Motherhood in itself is not degrading. Quite the opposite, it can be empowering, ecstatic, life and love-giving.

It is what society makes of it, and how it treats us, that makes it degrading. In our society we worry when there is a gap in our CV that says 'full-time mother' because others think it means we 'did nothing'. We need a society in which 'full-time mother' represents organisational skills, prioritising others, resilience and resourcefulness, multi-tasking, people management, and money management. 'Full-time mother' should be honoured and rewarded. If this were true, when we became mothers our status would increase.

8. *The need for competence and achievement.* Striving towards something, and feeling the joy of learning and being challenged, comes into this category. Being a new parent is a learning process and it is certainly a challenge. However, if we expect to be brilliant at it right from the start, then the joy of learning becomes fraught with fear. It is easy to take the challenge too far, especially if we have been particularly independent or successful in the past. Rising to a challenge, while having unrealistic expectations, can stop us from being able to receive or ask for help. Because society seems to expect mothers to just get on with it, without help, support, or praise, it is easy for new mums to expect too much of themselves. Being a new parent is a learning process, and this means that we will do it badly at times, or need to be mentored or helped at other times. Once we view new parenthood as a learning process, which needs help and support from others, it can be great fun to allow ourselves to enjoy the journey of learning, which includes getting it wrong, and getting help from others as we go along.

9. *The need for meaning and purpose.* This area of our lives gives us a reason to be here, and a reason to continue the struggle, even when it seems to be against the odds. When

our need for meaning and purpose is met, we are more resilient, and stronger in the face of adversity. When we have babies, the need for meaning and purpose is often met at a deep level. In our secular society, where there once was religion to fulfil the need for meaning and purpose, there is now often a void. However, having a baby can fill that void to some extent. There is a sense of purpose to your life now. Your reason for being here is to look after your baby and bring them up as best as you can. I have heard, countless times, from parents who are depressed, that the only reason they didn't take their own life was because of their children. Their children give them a reason to keep going when the going gets tough. Although having children can be the trigger that leads to depression, it is certainly also the case that having children can help us get through depression and come out the other side.

Did you think about which of these are most pertinent to perinatal depression? We are at risk of a reduction in *almost all* of these emotional needs when a baby arrives, apart from the need for meaning and purpose. Thinking about which are important for you, and which ones are not being met, can be a really useful exercise. Once you establish which ones are missing, you are halfway to rectifying the problem and reclaiming your health.

Depression is nature's call for help

There is also a theory that depression evolved as a call for help from the 'village'. If you live in a fairly small group of 50 to 100 people – the conditions in which our current brains are likely to have evolved – and you begin to feel depressed, the result may have been that the villagers helped to give you what you needed. If it was rest, they would do things for you. If it was attention or loving care, you would get attention or loving care. If it was encouragement to get back into doing things, you would get support, and so on. They would rally round and help sort the problem out. Today, in our overpopulated cities and private, enclosed houses, there is less support from our neighbours and community. We rely on our GP and health visitors, and this often isn't enough to lift us out of a bad patch, given that it involves a ten-minute meeting, after which you go back to an empty house. Having said that, the GP is important in that he or she can help ensure that you get some rest, by writing a sick note. Unfortunately, when you have a baby it is much harder for them to tell you to stop working, go to bed, and recover.

Depression is caused by lack of sleep

We have always known that disrupted sleep and depression go hand in hand. We used to think that depression causes sleep problems. However, new research is starting to show us that it may well be the other way around. It may well be that lack of sleep leads to anxiety and depression. Just read that again, and take in the enormity of that possibility: *it may well be that lack of sleep leads to depression*. If that is true, then no wonder perinatal depression is so common. No wonder men are also beginning to suffer from it, as they take a larger role in night-time wakings.

While we are still struggling to understand the mechanism and function of sleep, it does appear to have a role in 'processing' our emotions from the day before. While we sleep, we put to rest the challenges and uncertainties of the day before, clearing the way for fresh challenges for the next day. This is a process that involves the amygdala (which is our alarm system, reacting automatically when there is a problem or danger) and the prefrontal cortex (our rational,

77

calming system, which tells the amygdala that all is well). The research seems to suggest that communication between these two parts of the brain does not function well when we are sleep-deprived, and the amygdala stops 'listening' to the rational system. It just begins to run amok with fears and anxieties and worries, escalating into an irrational, illogical state of negativity and fear.

The Human Givens Institute has always maintained that sleep disruption causes depression. Traditionally, we have thought that when people are in poverty, or abusive relationships, or have lost a loved one, or are down on their luck, the added stress will affect their sleep, which can in turn lead to depression. This new research shows us that *all* you need is disrupted sleep to create a stress reaction. All you need to do is deprive a group of young people of their sleep for a number of days, and their brains' ability to regulate stress and negative emotion becomes temporarily damaged. Wow. Getting sleep is very important for a new parent. Being in a culture that prioritises the new mum's welfare, including the need for her to rest, sleep and eat, makes a lot of sense. Our culture sends new parents home within a few hours of giving birth, gives them responsibility for the welfare of their baby and the upkeep of the house, and feeding themselves, when they may have already missed two nights of sleep during the birth itself. Well, that is a recipe for depression.

Depression is caused by dietary factors

Your body is a machine that is so complicated that science has not yet managed to replicate its functions. It relies on food and drink to survive. It also relies on a range of nutrients and vitamins to keep all the aspects of your body working properly. Without vitamins and minerals, our bodies falter.

Research is beginning to show us that without certain vitamins and minerals, our brain chemistry falters too. And when our brain chemistry falters, we experience emotional problems as a consequence. For example, zinc, tryptophan and the B vitamins are necessary for the production of essential chemicals in the brain such as serotonin. A deficiency of serotonin has been linked to depression, and certain antidepressants are designed to remedy the serotonin imbalance. There has long been a link between coeliac disease and depression, in that the incidence of depression is much higher among people with this digestive problem. One theory is that the body is less able to digest the essential nutrients needed to keep the brain functioning at an optimum level. There is also growing evidence to suggest that, while 1 per cent of the population have coeliac disease, about five times that number have gluten sensitivity, which can also lead to psychiatric symptoms, including depression. However, it is not often the case that a GP will investigate the possibility of nutritional deficiencies in depression. They are much more likely just to prescribe antidepressants. I have heard of many profound and complete recoveries from depression just by avoiding wheat.

Other supplements which are linked with healthy brain function include omega-3 fatty acids, most commonly found in fish oils. Increasingly, research is showing us how important this special oil is in keeping brain function healthy. However, it may also be that it is beneficial in warding off depression. In some cases, it has even been shown to be as effective as antidepressants for treating depression (Lespérance and colleagues, 2010). While supplementing, or eating lots of fish and walnuts may be good for us, we do need to balance this with eating fewer omega-6 oils. These block the benefit of omega-3 oils. In our society of industrialised foods, we are eating an awful lot of omega-6 oils. They are found in biscuits, processed foods, breads, cakes, fast foods, ready-made meals and even in 'healthy' bottled salad dressings. Could it be that our modern diets are fuelling (excuse the pun) the burgeoning rates of depression in our culture?

Even with the evidence suggesting that omega-3s may help maintain healthy brain function, and can even treat cases of depression, we don't really know why it does so. One plausible theory is linked to the ability of omega-3s to reduce inflammation in the body. Inflammation as a cause of depression is a new theory. It is a bit of a breakthrough in the quest to find out what causes depression.

Depression as a symptom of inflammation

There is a new theory that proposes that depression is not a discreet condition, but that it is a symptom of something else. This intriguing suggestion casts depression as a symptom of a low-grade, chronic inflammatory response in the body. When your body is dealing with a problem, such as an injury or a virus, the immune system fires up and creates an inflammatory response to deal with the offending problem. While this works really well in the short term, the immune system response can stay activated rather than die down. This can lead to chronic, low-grade inflammation. During an inflammatory reaction, chemicals called 'inflammatory cytokines' are produced. These inflammatory cytokines can lead to a wide variety of psychiatric and neurological symptoms which are identical to the defining characteristics of depression. They affect the brain and the gut, and we are finding that the two are closely connected. Numerous studies have linked unfavourable changes to the bacteria in the gut with major depressive disorder. Also, research has shown us that the use of antidepressants (particularly SSRIs) is associated with a reduction in the production of pro-inflammatory cytokines.

The really interesting thing is that the body's inflammatory system responds in the same way to *physical* assault as it does to *emotional* assault (Gerhardt). Your body does not know the difference between a physical hurt and an emotional hurt – it creates an inflammatory response to both! I love this new finding, because it finally explains why the physical and emotional are inextricably linked. It might also explain why depression seems to have so many causes: lack of exercise, poor diet, abusive parenting, lack of sleep, isolation, poverty, bereavement and so on. Could it be that physical trauma to the body, such as lack of sleep, exercise, and poor diet, triggers the inflammatory response, which creates symptoms of depression? Emotional trauma, such as childhood neglect, bereavement, poverty, isolation and stress, could also trigger the inflammatory response, creating symptoms of depression.

The basic reason why we suffer mental problems is that brain and body are trying to 'save and protect' us from perceived danger. All the emotions that we feel so readily, but dislike so much, such as anger, jealousy, sadness, depression, anxiety, shame, and guilt, evolved for a reason. They are there to get us out of trouble. Danger for humans isn't just about saving us from tigers in the jungle, like it is for rabbits. Humans have very complicated and sophisticated brains that are highly socially evolved, and with that we also have a 'self-protection' kit, which activates very quickly and easily when there are stressors about. When we are stressed, our minds and bodies flip into 'emergency mode' very quickly, we release adrenalin and cortisol, which lead to a whole host of crazy, unstoppable reactions. We stop thinking straight, we over-react, we rubbish ourselves, we get angry with others, we feel sorry for ourselves, we think others are judging us, we feel inadequate and so on. This is not your fault: it is your brain trying to 'see' danger, and trying to 'react quickly' to protect you. It does this because of things that have happened in the past, and because of how our brains are wired. Let me give you an example. You might have been bitten by a dog as a child. Every time you see another dog, your brain jumps to your defence by making you scared, so you avoid the dog. You might know logically that the dog won't harm you, but you still feel scared, because your brain has taken over and is being scared for you to protect you.

Rather than trying to stop this happening, or berating ourselves because it happens, we could do with respecting this part of our brain that is working so hard to protect us, even though it is getting it wrong. Your brain doesn't realise that you don't need it to jump to your defence, or jump into attack mode. You can't fight it, you can't ignore it. The first step is to acknowledge and respect it for what it is. It is part and parcel of being a human.

However, there are ways of reducing the impact of your fight or flight system. We know that anyone can learn to reverse the process with practice, helping the body to switch from 'emergency' mode to 'everything is okay' mode. You do this by switching off the adrenalin response, and activating the relaxation response, or the 'calm and connect' system (which has been researched by Kerstin Uvnäs Moberg). The next chapter will give you lots of ways to do this. It doesn't always matter *why* you are depressed. If you can take care of yourself and help your body to release fewer stress hormones, it will have a beneficial effect on your mental state.

I hope that this whistle-stop tour of just a few of the current theories of what causes depression has given you an insight into how complicated the subject matter is, and shown that there doesn't seem to be one single cause of depression. The causes of depression lie in our biology, our physiology, our endocrine system, our neurology, our psychology, our social-psychology, our sociology, our culture and our evolutionary heritage. We will be taking a closer look at how you can help yourself in the next chapter. But we before we do that, it is worth just asking the question: could it be something else?

Could this be something other than depression?

You have had a baby. You are having trouble sleeping. You feel miserable, you are irritable, you don't feel yourself at all, and you are struggling to cope. This could be depression. However, it could also be something else. In order to find the right treatment, it is important to get the right diagnosis. So, before you or your doctor presumes that you have perinatal depression, it might be worth ruling out the following:

Postpartum thyroiditis

This is a rare complication that can develop after your baby is born. It can be diagnosed by your doctor with a blood test. The symptoms of postnatal thyroiditis can be very similar to those of depression and anxiety, and include fatigue, insomnia, palpitations, and irritability.

Trauma

It is becoming apparent that between 2 and 5 per cent of men and women end up with post-traumatic stress disorder (PTSD), and many more suffer acute stress disorder (ASD), as a result of their birth experience. ASD and PTSD are *psychological injuries* arising from traumatic experiences. They are not the same as a horrible birth experience. It is about what state the birth left you in, psychologically.

To use an analogy, it's like breaking a bone. I might fall down a big flight of stairs and walk away unscathed. On the other hand, I might trip up over nothing and break my ankle. I cannot predict this, or control it. If I have broken my ankle I am not weaker or more stupid than anyone else, and I cannot 'pull myself together'. I am injured, and I am unlucky. Sure, the level of the incident will have a part to play in the chance of being injured. If you fall off a cliff, you are more likely to have serious injuries. If your family is raped and murdered in front of your eyes, you are more likely to have serious psychological injuries. Also, if I had a former weakness in my ankle, I am more likely to re-injure it when I trip up. This follows for psychological injury too. For example, if you have an injection phobia, you *might be* more vulnerable to developing PTSD when you have a baby. Or if you were sexually assaulted as a child, you might be more vulnerable to trauma when you have your baby as an adult. Just as with depression, we are not absolutely sure what happens when we are traumatised, but we can recognise it and treat it.

What is birth trauma?

People who are traumatised will experience very unpleasant 'intrusions'. These can include nightmares, flashbacks, sudden fear, weepiness or panic attacks. Because these come out of the blue, they can be very disruptive, leaving you feeling agitated, insecure, scared, irritable, unable to sleep and lost. It is normal to feel like this for a few days or weeks after a traumatic event, while the brain sorts out what happened and commits it to memory. This is an unconscious process, in the same way as digestion is unconscious. However, when we develop PTSD, the brain has problems doing the processing and the event does not get committed to memory. It feels like it happened yesterday. Even as time passes, you still feel scared, as though it is still happening, or could happen again at any moment. Don't forget, this is not logical. You can't control this process logically. Because it feels so scary and horrible, you do your best to put it to the back of your mind, and avoid anything that makes you feel bad. You might push reminders of the event away, by avoiding television programmes, avoiding new babies, avoiding getting pregnant again, never talking about your birth, changing the subject as soon as you feel upset and so on. Psychologists call this 'avoidance' and it is a hallmark of PTSD. The more you push it away, the more your brain tries to bring it back so that it can heal (perhaps in the form of nightmares) and the more scared you feel, so you push it away…

So, if you are experiencing the following, it might be worth considering PTSD:

- Feeling as though it happened only yesterday, when the birth was more than three months ago
- Not being able to talk about it without crying, even though it happened more than three months ago
- If you were asked to tell someone about what happened in detail, or write it down in detail, you would be scared to do so
- Avoiding any reminders of what happened, because they make you feel bad
- You try to shove it to the back of your mind, but it keeps coming back
- Feeling generally anxious, tearful, irritable or as if you have changed as a person

If you explained the above to your GP, the chances are that

he or she would diagnose postnatal depression. This is not uncommon. Not only are the symptoms similar, but PTSD can cause depression. So often, we are suffering from both at the same time. A lot of PTSD is missed in postnatal women, and is labelled as postnatal depression. This matters, because the psychological treatments for postnatal depression and for PTSD are very different.

Notice that when diagnosing PTSD we emphasise that the initial trauma happened more than three months ago. Within that time, your mind and body might still be healing naturally, processing the event and committing it to memory, even if it is taking longer than you would like. You might meet the criteria for ASD, but the chances are you will get better. If you are talking to people about it, or crying and having nightmares, this is all part of the healing process. Keep doing those things. You might also try writing it all down in detail, or drawing pictures of how it felt, to help your brain process it. If you are going to do this, look after yourself while you do it. It can be hard going, and you need some tender loving care while you do this to keep you strong.

If it has been more than three months since the trauma, it may be that you are suffering from PTSD. Your brain carries on behaving as if you are still in danger (your anxiety levels remain high), and the brain seems to be trying to process it, but it can't. This is not your fault. It is just bad luck. However, it is very treatable.

Anxiety

Like PTSD and depression, anxiety and depression also go hand in hand. In cases of depression, anxiety and trauma, the 'fight/flight/freeze' part of the brain is being over-activated. Anxiety is often accompanied by unpleasant

---

Case study

Charlie got pregnant at the age of 28. She and her husband of four years had planned the pregnancy, and were excited and pleased. However, after she had had the baby, things weren't going so well. She was having problems sleeping. Whenever she tried to sleep, she would struggle to relax enough to be able to drop off. If she did manage to sleep, she would often wake up in a state of anxiety, because the baby had woken, but sometimes the baby would still be asleep. She was exhausted. She kept crying. She cried when she was alone, she cried when her husband came in from work. She also seemed to be irritable and angry at her husband all the time. She felt that people didn't understand. They said that she had changed, and she knew they were right. She had changed. She had known that having a baby can be hard. But she hadn't expected it to be this hard. She didn't feel any love for her baby. In fact, when she looked at her baby she felt resentment. She felt confused and hopeless, and she felt awful because she was not enjoying motherhood. Under pressure from her family, she went to her GP for help.

---

physical symptoms such as heart racing, stomach churning, feeling hot and sweaty and being unable to stay still. Anxiety also has an effect on the mind, in that you will be hyper-vigilant, aware of potential dangers, unable to sleep, jumpy and always thinking the worst. Behaviourally, anxiety can make you rush around like a gerbil on a treadmill, always on the go, always restless, drinking far too much tea and coffee, eating sugar-rich foods, and not realising that you are exhausting yourself. If someone tells you to take a break and rest, you can't. As Kate put it, 'I literally did everything, all the time and I was exhausted. I was extremely irritable but I felt like I couldn't sit down and relax. In all honesty having a baby sent me doolally, and my anxiety was through the roof'.

Bipolar depression

Bipolar depression used to be known as manic depression. With unipolar depression, as described above, the sufferer has episodes of feeling incredibly down, fed up, lacking in energy and so on. However, with bipolar depression, the moods don't just flip from normal to depressed, they flip from super-hyped, down to depressed and back again. When she is 'manic' the sufferer might feel elated, energised, excited, and throw caution to the wind, not need to sleep, not need to eat, do things to the extreme, such as shop, socialise, clean, gamble, and so on. The extremes can make life very difficult. Spending too much money, not sleeping properly, gambling, drinking too much, taking on big projects, never resting and so on, makes for an exhausted person who then collapses in a heap of depression. Bipolar can fool us, because we can be extremely happy and energetic, but there is still something wrong with our ability to regulate our mood. Bipolar depression tends to show itself before pregnancy, so if you know you are vulnerable to it, you can build in a plan for managing it when your baby arrives.

Obsessional Compulsive Disorder (OCD)

OCD is a form of anxiety. Research shows that pregnancy and birth are common triggers for this distressing disorder, which has led to the new term 'perinatal OCD', or 'maternal OCD'. It makes sense that pregnancy and birth can trigger episodes of OCD, because OCD is all about feeling anxious and trying to stay safe. Keeping baby safe is a concern for many parents. Even *before* we become pregnant, we are bombarded with information about which supplements we should be taking. Given the common health scares that we are fed in the media, and the fact that our culture leaves mum and dad alone with the baby, inexperienced and unsure, practically from birth, it is not surprising that being anxious about safety is a common problem perinatally. Even if the new parents have the benefit of an older relative to hand, who has been there and done that before, their 'advice' will be out of date compared to the current guidelines. So, carrying a baby in utero, and bringing a new baby home, is scarier than it would be in other cultures, or in times gone by. The irony is that babies are actually safer than they ever were before, but our anxiety seems to be much greater.

There are two main hallmarks of perinatal OCD. The 'obsessional' component involves distressing thoughts and imagining harm coming to your baby. The key word here is 'distressing'. When these images pop into your mind, they upset you. A common one is seeing images of you throwing your own baby down the stairs. Because the images or thoughts are so distressing, they are followed by a 'compulsion' to put it right. This can take many forms. The compulsions can be physical, such as going to check that your baby is okay, or washing your hands, or asking your partner for reassurance that you aren't going mad. The compulsion can be a thought, such as counting to fifty, or praying, or quickly thinking about something else. The more that the distressing thoughts come, the more compelled you feel to put it right. So you get into a habit of needing to do the compulsions to feel better, but rather than feeling better, you get into a vicious cycle of constantly having to do the compulsions to avoid strong anxiety. Once the habit has got hold, there's no stopping the vicious cycle, and you can find yourself spending hours each day in compulsive behaviour, leaving you exhausted and frightened. It is like an addiction, but with no good feelings. The worst thing about perinatal OCD is that the mother often feels deeply ashamed of her thoughts, believing that they make her a bad mother. Ironically, it is because she is exactly the type of person who is *nothing* like her disturbing thoughts, that the thoughts have the power to upset her so much. So, while she may be scared that she is going to harm her baby, we know that the very fact that she is so horrified by that thought makes her a safe mother, and one who is not a danger to her baby. If you think you might be suffering from perinatal OCD, I'll say it for you again: the very fact that you get horrible images and thoughts of harming your baby, and that they distress you, tells us that you are not going to harm your baby.

As well as fearing that she might harm her baby, a mother with OCD may also fear that she is going mad. This can be very scary and deeply unpleasant. Once again, I would like to reassure you that if you think you might be going mad, *you are not going mad*. True madness (or psychosis, as the professionals term it) comes when we have lost complete touch with reality, and have no idea that we are behaving in an odd or strange way. Eve Canavan writes about her experience of surviving postnatal psychosis (along with severe anxiety) very succinctly. She describes how she lost touch with reality. 'I remember the terror very well. But they also seemed logical. I would say to John "I'm trapped in motherhood... I'm trapped in the world John. And the clouds, they are getting closer everyday. I need to climb the tree and cut them with scissors and then I'll get to space. But what will I do when I'm there?"' As you can see when you read this example, madness is something other people are aware of, because you make no sense to them. But to the psychotic person, it all seems to be logical and make absolute sense. So, if you are in touch with reality enough to know that your feelings and behaviours are odd, then you are not going mad. (By the way, if someone you love has just had a baby, and is saying meaningless things like the above, and they don't seem to realise it, please seek advice, as this form of behaviour can be a sign of puerperal psychosis, which can be quite serious.)

What is normal?

Having read about some of the mental health problems that are possible perinatally, it would be natural for you to now be thinking 'Oh my goodness, I've got postnatal depression, OCD, trauma…' and so on. However, all mental health problems are on a continuum, and all people have difficult thoughts and feelings to contend with. Please just read that again. *All people have difficult thoughts and feelings to contend with.* It comes with being human. When you have had a baby, there will be some or all of these difficult, unpleasant, confusing, horrible feelings in the mix. You have never done this before, you are quickly having to learn to do things you've never had to do before, you are responsible for a new life, you don't know if you're doing it 'right' or not, and so on. Also, nature has arranged it so that you are more 'wired' and alert to danger (presumably so that you can protect your baby). The mothering hormone prolactin is responsible for this. You might find it really difficult to leave the house with your baby, because it doesn't feel safe. Or you might find it difficult to sleep because you feel you need to watch your baby sleep in case something happens. You are constantly checking things, constantly talking about and thinking about your baby, constantly in a mild state of worry and unease. Accepting this as a normal part of the tapestry of new parenthood is part of the journey. So, if you find that you are more worried or tearful than usual, go easy on yourself and remember that you are doing something very difficult and pretty amazing. Babies catapult us into a world of strong feelings that we've never had before. Don't fight them. Go with them. While it is natural to feel some anxiety about being a new parent, it is not natural to *suffer*. If you feel it is getting in the way of things, making you miserable, or stopping you from leading a normal life, then tell someone. However, do allow yourself to feel sorry for yourself, to feel anxious, to feel like you are slightly crazy at times, to feel inadequate, to feel sad and so on. We all feel these things, and they are what make us human. You can't have sunshine without a little bit of rain. But the rain should always stop now and again, and let the sun come out.

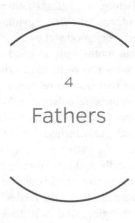

4

Fathers

The world is changing fast. In my lifetime, we have moved from a world where fathers go out to work, and mothers stay at home to look after the children and house, to one where mothers and fathers both go out to work and both stay at home to look after the children and house. Along with this change have come revisions to attitudes and assumptions about gender differences. Expectations of women in the workplace have changed dramatically. Women are now willing and able to hold positions that were traditionally reserved for men, such as soldiers, firefighters, CEOs, managers and so on. However, there has been an equally great corresponding shift for men. This has happened not in the workplace, but at home. Men are now willing and able to take a much wider role within the home. They are now caregivers, birth companions, nappy changers, nurturers, counsellors: hands-on parents. Research is exploring what fathers have to offer in ways that it never has before. We are learning that fathers matter to the development of the baby and child in the same way that mothers do. This is surprising us. Before, we thought fathers were important in supporting mothers, and in providing discipline. We thought they weren't very good at the nurturing side of things, because that is what mothers are so good at. After all, it's in their biology. It's what we see in most other mammals. We focused on the fact that women release oxytocin when they birth and when they breastfeed. Not men. We saw that women have strong emotional bonds with their babies, whereas men can be more rational and detached. We believed that women find it easier to have the patience and warmth that children need. It comes naturally to them. Women can multitask. It is what we see in nature – the mothers do the loving, attaching, parenting thing. Very few males do. And so on.

But things are changing. And as attitudes change, so does the science. Scientists are now asking questions such as 'What happens to men's hormones when they hear a baby cry?' and 'How do babies respond to their fathers' faces?' and 'What happens to children when fathers are not emotionally available?' and so on. And because we are actually asking those questions, we are learning that fathers have many similarities to mothers.

You have a parenting hormone kit too

Oxytocin is one of the hormones that facilitates love, attachment, bonding, trust and co-dependency. It is released when people who love each other kiss, cuddle, make eye contact, and even when they eat together! This gives a romantic dinner a whole new meaning. We know that mothers and babies release oxytocin at birth, which has an obvious evolutionary function of helping them connect and get to know each other. (Let's face it, without the natural glue of oxytocin, a mother is quite likely to decide to walk away from that wet, blue, limp-looking thing that she pushed out of her nether regions!). It was long thought that bonding between dads and babies happens later, and more slowly than it seems to with mums and babies. And this was probably because it was true. Mums sometimes fall in love quite quickly and quite ferociously with their babies, and dads are left feeling bewildered at this phenomenon, feeling less than enamoured with the strange looking creature that seems to do very little but poo and cry.

But this is changing. Men's hormones are changing. Men's behaviour is changing. Men's brain chemistry is changing. Why? It might be because of the way they behave. Science is showing us that certain behaviours trigger hormonal changes, as well as vice versa. Let me illustrate this with an example.

Birth 100 years ago

Typically, the mother labours upstairs in her home, with womenfolk around. There is peace, quiet, and safe, trusted attendants. There is no medical equipment or chemical/synthetic oxytocin, so she births her baby using her own natural oxytocin. The father is downstairs. He does not see the process. He helps by providing towels and water. When the baby is born, the mother stays in 'confinement' while she adapts to breastfeeding her infant and recovers. Breastfeeding leads to more release of oxytocin. Father carries on as usual. He shows little interest in the moment-by-moment behaviours or needs of his child, although he feels fiercely proud and protective. The mother's oxytocin levels are high, the father's oxytocin levels are not.

Birth 50 years ago

Mothers have been moved into hospitals to birth, and the system has become medicalised. She feels unsupported, alone and frightened. She is offered more medication, and more women birth their babies with chemical or physical assistance. She produces less natural oxytocin at birth. Her baby is removed and dressed and put in a nursery, and she is encouraged to bottle-feed because it is more 'sterile'. She is producing a lot less natural oxytocin than the previous generation. Fathers are still outside the birthing room; their hormone production is arguably no different. Mothers are beginning to say that they want fathers with them, because they feel frightened and alone.

Birth 10 years ago

Fathers are with mothers for the birth. They stay in the room throughout the process. They are witness to their baby being born. They see their partner labour, they hold her, support her, feed her and nurture her. They see the incredible birth of their newborn baby, and they hold their newborn within minutes of the birth. They look into their baby's eyes. They are encouraged to take their shirt off and hold their baby close, skin-to-skin. They talk to their baby, and they notice that their baby looks up. Magic happens and dads fall in love with their babies very quickly indeed. Their oxytocin levels are through the roof!

Research is showing us that when a father is expecting a baby, there are some incredible changes happening for him, as well as for the mother. Hormonal changes take place, such as a reduction in testosterone and increases in prolactin, oxytocin and vasopressin. These prepare him for the gentle, loving, strong role of fatherhood and family bonding. Vasopressin is particularly pertinent for dads, as it has a more powerful impact on fathers than it does on mothers. Vasopressin has been referred to as the 'monogamy' hormone, as it reduces sexual drive, increases protection and dedication towards family, and promotes bonding and familial connectedness. As Theresa Crenshaw puts it 'Testosterone wants to prowl, vasopressin wants to stay home'. Other examples of the changes that take place when a man is expecting a baby include the fact that men get better at hearing a baby's cry as the due date approaches. Feldman found that fathers' oxytocin levels rise before the birth, and continue to rise and fall according to how much he interacts with his baby, and also in rhythm with the mother's levels of oxytocin. The more time he spends with his baby and his family, the more his hormones and brain chemistry adapt accordingly. This is not just true for humans. It is also true for rats. Male rats demonstrate changes in the brain within days of the pups being born. However, this only happens if the male rat is kept in proximity to the pups. The very *act* of fathering releases the relevant hormonal and biochemical orchestration. These hormones have a direct impact on brain functioning (directing which parts of the brain are activated) and they have a direct behavioural and emotional impact too. They change how we feel and what we do. So, for example, in one study oxytocin (when inhaled) was shown to increase the amount that fathers smiled, looked at, laughed with and interacted with their babies (this was compared to a group of fathers who were not given oxytocin, but were given a placebo). Even more interestingly, the level of oxytocin in the dad had an immediate and direct impact on the babies. The babies' levels of smiling, laughing, eye contact and playfulness also increased in response to their dad's behaviour.

Dads, you matter to your children. We have known this for a long time. Children who have been raised without a father are more likely to experience emotional difficulties, and get into trouble with the law (please look back at the section about research, evidence and statistics on page 32) This tells us nothing about *your* child, given that there are so many other variables that can impact on a child's life. It is a statistic, a generality, not information about your situation, or your neighbour's situation, or anyone else's situation). The fact that an absent father can impact negatively on a child's emotional state is something that I have, in the past, put down to social factors. One-parent families are more likely to struggle in general, through poverty, social denigration, stigma and so on. However, it seems that it may not be only a social issue. Going back to the example of rats, it would seem that for Degu rats, removing fathers from the litter leads to dramatic changes in the brains of the pups. Degu rats share the parenting role. The fathers spend the first few days helping with the basic care such as nesting, warming and grooming. Then, as the pups get older, the fathers begin to actively play with the youngsters. In experimental situations where the father was removed from the Degu litter, researchers found that the brain development of the pups was different from those whose fathers stayed with the litter. In effect, there was brain damage to the pups without a father, in terms of fewer synapses in the parts of the brain responsible for regulating emotion and reward. While we can't extrapolate directly from rats to humans, this is still interesting research. Having an involved father around while you are growing up may be good for your brain development, and in particular your ability to regulate emotion. Fathers matter.

Overall, as things are changing, we are realising that mums and dads both have the propensity to be amazing parents. Dads can't gestate or birth babies, but they can do everything else. They can release the 'parenting' hormones of vasopressin, prolactin and oxytocin. They can suppress their aggression by reducing testosterone release. They can even lactate. (Yes, you read that right. All mammals can lactate in theory. You don't need a full breast, you just need a nipple, a pituitary gland and the right cocktail of hormones. Humans are not the only mammals where the male can lactate. Male bats, goats and guinea pigs have been known to do so, among others. In some pygmy cultures, men have been seen nursing infants as part of their parental role). Dads, you rock! And the more you partake in parenting, the more you release the right hormones to facilitate your daddy role, such as falling in love with your baby, nurturing your baby, being sensitive to your baby, sharing joy with your baby, and being important to, and responded to, by your baby.

Dads and perinatal depression

As fathers become more and more involved in the preparations for the baby, in home life, and in caring for the baby, it would seem that they might be paying the same price that women pay. The number of men diagnosed with perinatal depression seems to be on the increase. If you are a man who is going to become a father, or has just become a father, and you are struggling emotionally, then you are not alone. Estimates range from 1 in 10 to 1 in 4 new fathers experiencing perinatal depression. That is as high as some of the estimates for new mothers.

Is it definitely the case that depression is on the increase for expectant fathers? It might be that men have always experienced perinatal depression, but that they expressed this in a different way. It has long been known that men are less likely to seek help from their GP, for example. They are more likely to keep their distress to themselves, or to express it in the use of alcohol or anger and aggression. So, it may be that men have always experienced perinatal depression, but that we just didn't know about it.

So men may hide their emotional suffering in ways that women don't, by not going to the GP. And researchers may have not noticed the prevalence of paternal depression because they didn't think to ask the question. However, it may well be the case that paternal depression is actually on the increase, simply because being a parent is hard, and men are parenting more than they were before. They are sharing the same struggles as women, such as responsibility, change, isolation, and lack of a supportive 'village' or wise elders.

However, there are specific issues for men and boys brought about by our societal expectations. And at the moment, men's roles are in such dramatic flux that it is difficult to see the wood for the trees.

There have been such dramatic changes in societal beliefs and expectations of women in the past 100 years. Only just over 100 years ago, women were viewed as too weak to exercise, too stupid to vote, and needing to be disciplined by their man in order to ensure subservience. While feminism brought dramatic changes to what is expected of womanhood, it has left a bit of a void around what to expect of men. Our society is in the process of brushing off the old rigid masculine expectations such as needing to be aggressive, emotionally distant and the sole provider. But what replaces them? Well, I think this is rather exciting, because I think what replaces them is emotional intelligence – the ability to be aware of and in tune with your own emotions and those of others, and to be able to use those emotions to negotiate life and relationships effectively. Whereas men used to be encouraged to be emotionally cut-off from their feelings, we are now raising men to be more emotionally attuned, aware of the needs of themselves and others, and able to verbalise those feelings and meet those needs. They are emotionally mature and self-aware. Men as parents need to begin to state their needs, and find ways of expressing them and meeting them, so that they can connect in increasingly meaningful and powerful ways to their children and babies. All humans have a need to be connected with their family, to feel wanted, important and relevant. Steve Biddulph argues that in most societies, this is not a problem for men. This is because in most societies, the place where a man works is also the place where he plays, rests and connects. It is home. If his tasks take him away from home, he takes a child or two with him, as a part of their learning and development. He is a constant role model, constantly a part of the family. However, with the onset of industrialisation, men were physically removed from their homes to a separate place of work, for most of the child's waking day. In order to facilitate this, society created an expectation that men be emotionally cut-off, tough and aggressive. Biddulph refers to this as a deep 'wound' that we now need to begin to heal. To do so, we need to pay attention to men's needs and help them to be loving, connected dads who really belong back in the heart of the family. Because men in our very recent cultural history were out of the house most of the time, and when they came home they were only expected to tell their children off, we have got into a situation whereby 'We men want to be good dads, when most of us have never seen what a good dad looks like' (Biddulph, *Juno* magazine).

There is a risk that we are casting men back into the family (insisting that they be at the birth, that they change nappies, that they bath the children after a full day's work, that they be a shoulder for mum to cry on, and so on) without paying attention to their needs in the process, because society has forgotten that men feel emotional pain too. Men, we need to honour you, your masculinity, your importance in your children's lives, and your emotional needs. However, in respecting your emotional needs, we don't want to infantilise or patronise you. As Biddulph puts it 'There's no place here for the man who wants to be the centre of attention – a trait that only looks good on a baby, and baby-men really don't cut the mustard in the husband stakes. What is needed is self-sufficiency, a willingness to trust that your partner will come back to you when mouths have been fed and needs met, and to be appealing as a steady and fun and nurturing adult partner'. Thus, while we are asking a lot more of our men in terms of physical demands, we are also asking a lot more in terms of emotional maturity. To be able to be more emotionally mature, or emotionally intelligent, we need you to find a voice in the parenting sphere. There are some aspects of fathering that have not got a real voice, in that you can't really get a handle on what you might feel, what you might expect to feel, what is okay and what isn't. Let's begin by considering your presence at the birth.

Fathers at the birth of their baby

Cross-culturally and traditionally, birthing was the realm of women. Even when male doctors began to get involved in the late Middle Ages, it was only the medics that were present. Fathers stayed outside the birthing room. They might be helpful in terms of providing hot water and towels, but they did not attend the birth itself. They stayed downstairs. When birth moved into hospitals, men had to pace the corridor, outside the birthing room, because they were not allowed in (just for fun, did you know that you were considered a 'bio hazard'?) You were invited in when the mother was presentable, and when baby was wrapped and bathed. Of course, some men are intrigued by nature's miracle in action, and some men in medieval times would illegally find ways to sneak into the birthing room out of sheer fascination. Some fathers today are mesmerised, and fall in love even more with their partners for being so amazing. They can't wait to see their baby's head and body emerge, fully in awe of nature and her powers, and not in the least bit fazed by wetness, goo, and some ickiness.

However, some men find it very difficult to be at the birth of their baby. They find it difficult to see their partner in pain, as they don't understand that the pain is different to dental pain or having your fingernails pulled out. They find it difficult to not be scared, because they've heard that birth can be dangerous. They find it difficult to see the blood and goo and poo, and especially to see her pretty labia so (temporarily) altered. But do you have a voice to share this? Not really. There is a lot of pressure on dads to attend the birth of their babies. If you share that you are anxious about being at the birth, at best, society won't hear you. At worst, you will be criticised for being thoughtless and selfish. That is what I mean when I say you haven't got a voice yet.

Staying with the example of being present at the birth, you have an added pressure. Sure, the mother needs to actually birth the baby, but did you ever consider that you are expected to be her emotional support through the epic journey that is labour and birth? At a hospital birth there's often no one else there! The midwife keeps coming in and out. If she stays in, she is busy with paperwork. The emotional support now comes from the father, not from the midwife, or the aunts and mothers. This is a great burden, and one that I think is too heavy for many fathers, simply because they are not very well prepared or supported to do this difficult job. I know how difficult it is, because I am a birth doula! Expecting fathers to always be at the birth is adding to the prevalence of postnatal mental health problems, because dads are coming out of the birthing room exhausted, traumatised and feeling guilty or inadequate.

You are then expected to go home and look after the house, the mum *and* the baby. Meanwhile, everyone pays attention to the mother and the baby, and sometimes they don't even ask you how you are. While everyone knows what the traumas of birth might have been for the woman, society hasn't yet begun to talk about the traumas for the birthing partner. If no one else can talk about it, how can you be expected to? The one support that you did have (your partner) is now emotionally tied up in her little baby, leaving you on the sidelines, trying to be a good enough support to her. That is not the best start to parenthood.

It might seem as if I am exaggerating these details to get my message across, but in fact, I think this issue is much bigger than I suggest. Michel Odent (a well-known obstetrician and natural birth guru) has long said that not only do fathers often make poor birth partners (because mothers feel self-conscious in their presence, and because dads bring too much adrenalin into the room), but also that it can be detrimental to the couple's sex life, because the man can find it difficult to see his partner in the same sexy light as he did before the birth. This is an area that is not talked about. How can men come to terms with how they are feeling, and what they are going through, if as a society we can't even talk about how they *might* feel? It is not politically correct to say that a man might find it difficult to resume sexual intimacy after birth. There is not the cultural language or understanding of what men might be feeling that there is for women. Men are simply expected to be at the birth (or they are heavily criticised for being selfish), and they are expected to witness it without proper preparation, and without any emotional repercussions. Women have many more avenues to express their birth trauma than men do, both in the form of physical support (such as support groups, NHS pathways and internet support) and in the form of people being able to listen and sympathise more readily, because they can understand that a woman can have an awful birth, but not a man.

If you are a man and you think you have been traumatised by being at your partner's birth, then you probably have. It is worth reading the section above on trauma (the symptoms are the same in women as they are in men) and finding a way through it. You are not alone, you are not bad, and you are not weak. You are responding normally to an abnormal event, and you may benefit from a little help to process the trauma and get yourself through to the other side. If you are a man who is going to be at the birth of your baby, then I suggest you prepare for the event, and think about your wishes at the birth, and not just those of your partner. Do you want extra support, for example from a doula or a relative? Do you want to see the baby's head emerging? Do you want to hold the baby skin-to-skin? If you are having doubts about being there at all, do share them and talk them through with someone. Your feelings matter too.

So, as I was saying, perinatal depression seems to be on the rise for men. In my view this is largely due to the changing role of fathers. Traditionally, the whole family would get involved in parenting. After all, it has only fairly recently become normal for a couple to be living on their own when they have their first baby. In other cultures, and not so long ago in our own culture, families would share houses across the generations, living with either their own parents or the in-laws. When you had a baby, you had other people in the house who had done it before. They could cook your tea, clean the house, or take the baby for a while and calm it. Nowadays it's all down to you! When mum is distressed, or struggling, or can't manage the cooking, or needs a shower, or can't calm the baby, you are the only one who can help. The family has been reduced down to you. Nowadays, couples *want* to be the only ones on this journey. They don't want others involved. While that is nice, it does leave a lot of pressure on the father, as he is the sole means of physical and emotional support. The pressure is even greater if you haven't done this before, or if you are trying to hold down a job at the same time, keeping a boss happy or running your own business. Anna Machin has studied fatherhood. As she puts it 'Men are where women were in the 1980s: they are told "you can have it all" and then suddenly discover they can't without experiencing a considerable negative impact on their physical and mental wellbeing [in the form of] feelings of guilt, deep disappointment and emotional pressure engendered by trying to juggle different elements of their life without any support'.

In conclusion, perinatal depression matters to fathers too. Many of the issues are the same for mums as they are for dads, including lack of support, previous history of depression, lack of sleep, loss of previous life, adjustment to change and so on. Both sexes commonly begin to feel depressed during the pregnancy, not just after the birth. Both sexes are more vulnerable when there is a lack of support, in the form of direct hands-on support, from family and health care staff, as well as emotional support in the form of checking in with fathers and mothers to see how they're doing, and reassuring them when they need it.

Men have some differing issues, related to differing societal expectations. Men are now the main emotional and practical support for the new mother, and I think this is an unrecognised pressure on fathers. And yet, at the same time as giving them this added role, we still expect them to resume a full-time job after two weeks, and to bring in the bacon as if nothing had happened. And men haven't yet got a narrative, or a voice, to help them make sense of their feelings. Most psychologists struggle to recruit volunteers for research, but when trying to understand what life is like for fathers, Machin had the opposite experience. 'Fathers want their voice heard. I was surprised that I had no problems recruiting men for this study – in fact it was massively oversubscribed'.

The bottom line is that in this self-sufficient society you need to take care of yourself, because no one else is going to do it for you. You, as a couple, matter. I have been at many births where the father is reluctant to take a break, or have something to eat, because he thinks he doesn't matter as much as his partner during the birth. In one case, I learnt my lesson when I had to stuff a biscuit in a father's mouth to stop him from passing out! Since then, I insist that dads look after themselves during the birth, before they even realise that they are in need of anything.

So, dads – all the tips, advice, techniques and information in this book are aimed at you too. Your job is to take care of your partner, so she can be strong for your baby. But to do that, you also need to take care of yourself in the process. Read all of this book – almost all of it applies to you too. Remember that on aeroplanes, adults are asked to put on their oxygen masks before helping the children. It is the same for fathers. Take care of yourself emotionally so that you can be strong enough to take care of your partner and your baby.

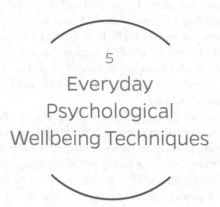

5
Everyday Psychological Wellbeing Techniques

When things are going well, we tend to just carry on with life, without necessarily taking any special care of ourselves. For example, we don't take care of our backs, until something happens. When things are going well, we will sit for long spells in poor positions, we won't spend money on the expensive supportive pillow, we won't book in a back massage. But when our back gives us problems, we begin to take care of it in the same way that we should have done all along. It is the same with our mental health. Here are some super techniques for psychological self-care that I would advise everyone to adhere to. Don't wait until your mind and body are crying out for it. Do it now, to protect yourself from future stressors and problems. All the techniques have the same benefit – they get your mind and body out of 'emergency' adrenalin mode, into 'calm and connect' mode.

Building a happy brain with mind exercises
Research shows us that positivity is good for our health. This

makes perfect sense. When we mull over negative things, watch negative programmes, or focus on how unfair our lives are, we actually feel worse. We are activating the part of our brain that is good at feeling rubbish – the emotional pain centres. What research is showing us, is that brain function works a bit like muscle function. When brains work, they develop neural pathways, just like when muscles work, they develop muscle fibres. If I work my arm a lot in a gym, it will get stronger, but my leg muscles won't. So I can choose which muscles I want to strengthen and build. It is the same with the brain. I can choose which parts of my brain I want to 'work on' by exercising those parts. I can choose to get really good at feeling hard done by, feeling sad for the world, or feeling angry at my sister, thereby exercising the emotional pain circuits of my brain. Alternatively, I can choose to exercise the joy and happiness parts of my brain. I would do this by focussing on the things in life that make me feel good, such as people I like being with, things I like doing, and/or things I am grateful for. Simple.

Research shows us that being optimistic is good for us. Those of us who are pessimistic seem to have practised and developed strong neural pathways that habitually presume 'I am never lucky, you don't get anything for nothing in this world, people are out to get you, life is unfair' and so on. Those of us who are optimistic, have practised and developed strong neural pathways that habitually presume 'life is great, people are friendly and kind, I am a lucky person, things always work out in the end' and so on. What is interesting is that these beliefs are self-fulfilling. If you believe you are lucky, you will be luckier than if you believe you are unlucky! Richard Wiseman has been researching optimism for many years. In one piece of research, people were divided up into those who believed themselves to be generally lucky people (the optimists) and those who believed themselves to be generally unlucky people (the pessimists). They were then all asked to flick through a newspaper and count how many photographs there were. What they didn't know was that within the newspaper, the following was written: 'Stop counting, tell the experimenter you have seen this and win $250.' On average, the self-reported lucky people spotted this and received their money. However, the self-reported unlucky people did not. Wiseman is clear that when we believe something, we behave in a way that fulfils that belief. So, if we believe we are unlucky, we actually bring about our own bad luck, and vice versa.

So, being optimistic is a great trait to have, and you can practise it by replacing negative thinking with more joyful thinking.

Here are some techniques that will help you to do that.

1. Affirmations

Affirmations are simply positive statements, repeated to yourself on a regular basis. They can be useful for consolidating existing beliefs, but they can also be used to change your mind-set into a more positive one. The evidence for whether affirmations actually work or not is inconclusive. It seems to be the case that affirmations can create chemical changes in the brain that can cement new ideas, feelings or associations. I know this, because I have used them and they make an enormous difference to me. However, they can make you feel worse. If you choose an affirmation that reminds you of something that makes you feel bad, then affirmations can reinforce the negativity. For example, if I have a facial disfigurement that I feel ashamed of, and I choose an affirmation that says 'I look beautiful', then the chances are that the affirmation just reminds me that I am facially disfigured, and I end up feeling worse. I would need to make it a little more realistic. It might be better to use 'My life is full and rewarding' or 'I use my smile to the best of my ability'. However, if I have a facial disfigurement that I have no shame about, that I accept and live in peace with, then the affirmation 'I am beautiful' could benefit me. To summarise, when using affirmations bear in mind that if you are particularly distressed their uses can be limited. And realism helps. Should you choose to use affirmations in your everyday life, here are some tips.

One of the best ways to use affirmations is to think about the things you are grateful for (this is best done on a good day). For example, 'I have a roof over my head'. 'I love visiting the Lakes'. 'I have full mobility, I can walk and run'. 'I am lucky to be a mother'. 'I enjoy cuddles'. 'I love my bed'. Don't write down what you *should* be grateful for, as this may trigger guilt. Then, think about all the things that are your strengths or qualities (if you can't think of any, then ask yourself what other people have said about your strengths and qualities). If you're feeling brave, put down the things that you *would like* to be your qualities, but you feel need a little work. For example, 'I listen well to people', 'I have a sense of humour', 'People like my company', 'I am good at music', 'I have kind eyes', 'I am a successful business woman', 'I try really hard to be the best mum I can be', 'I forgive myself when I am not perfect'. Write them down.

Once you have written them down, it is time to 'expose' yourself to them regularly. You can do this in a number of ways. Repetition is key. Just as advertising works best with repetition, so do affirmations. You can print them all out, and pin them up on your bathroom cabinet. You can write one in dry-wipe pen on your rear-view mirror, and change it every week. You can put one as a reminder on your phone, so it will 'ping up' at you once a day. You can put one on your kettle, so that each time you boil your kettle, you see it. You can write one in dry-wipe pen on your baby's feeding bottle or cup, if they have one. You get the gist. Use sticky notes, marker pens, phones or simple pen and paper. See the affirmations on a daily basis. In the end, they become part of your thinking, a part of who you are and what you believe.

2. Visualisation

Visualisation, or 'imagining' things, is a fast-track route to changing your emotions. I'll give you an example. When you read a novel, you might sit in the same chair, in the same room, in the same house, no matter which book you read. But you will feel very different, according to which book you read. It isn't your situation that changes how you feel, it is your imagination being sparked by the book. A scary book is likely to lead you to feel jumpy, jittery, nervous, and hyper-vigilant. When the cat miaows from behind you, you startle. A comedy is likely to have your tummy muscles twitching with mirth, and you may even laugh out loud, releasing all those lovely hormones associated with laughter. A sexy book will also help you release specific hormones that have nothing to do with your living room, and everything to do with your imagination! Your imagination has the power to trigger the release of specific chemicals in your body which affect how you feel. Relaxed or tense, angry or joyful, loved-up or hungry... your body can feel these in the absence of anything 'real' or physical.

You can learn to use visualisations to change what is happening in your body, and how you feel. It is so easy, and yet we don't do it. This is how easy it is.

In a moment, I want you to close your eyes, and take a deep breath in, and an even longer breath out, twice. I then want you to remember a time when you were relaxing on holiday, or relaxing in a favourite place in nature. Take yourself, in your mind's eye, back to that especially relaxing time. Imagine that you are there again. You can boost your imagination by focussing on four modalities: what you can see, hear, smell and feel. You might focus on the colours around you, the views. You might focus on what you can hear around you – the silence, the wind, the waves, people in the distance. You might focus on what you can smell – the smell of fresh air, or suntan lotion. You might focus on what you can feel on your skin – a breeze, the sun, leaves underfoot. Once you have decided what your special relaxing place is going to be, it is time to put this book down, get yourself comfortable, close your eyes, take in two long breaths and really go for it.

How was that? Did you notice that you feel more relaxed now than you did before? If so, you just managed to calm yourself physiologically, within minutes. With practice, this gets better and better, easier and easier and more and more effective. I'd advise you to practise on good days, so that when you need it on a bad day, it will help you. It's no good saving it for a bad day. Your stress is very unlikely to allow it to work unless you have practised it beforehand.

3. Mindfulness

Mindfulness is popular at the moment. Everyone is talking about it and it has become a staple technique in many therapies. Mindfulness is a wonderful tool for combatting both stress and depression. The beauty of mindfulness is that it doesn't try to change anything or fight anything. It just accepts things as they are. Acceptance is something that we struggle with when we are anxious or depressed. Many people talk about 'fighting' anxiety or 'combatting' depression. Research suggests that accepting it can be much more beneficial. After all, you are only human, and all humans have rubbish feelings such as anger, guilt, jealousy, inadequacy, hopelessness and inactivity. Let me repeat that. *All humans* feel rubbish quite a lot of the time! The other benefit of mindfulness is that it helps us to do something that humans are notoriously bad at – living in, and noticing, the present moment. Living in the present moment is associated with calm, relaxation, acceptance, gratitude and positivity. You might think you're quite good at this, but think again. When you last had a cup of tea, did you *notice* what it was like to sit and drink it? Did you notice what the tea felt like on your tongue? Did you *notice* how it felt when you swallowed the tea? What happened in the muscles of your throat and stomach? Do you even remember what it felt like to drink your cup of tea? Or did you mindlessly gulp it down while you were thinking of what you needed to do, or what happened last night? If you are thinking 'I couldn't focus on my tea, because I had a toddler climbing the fireplace that I needed to respond to,' then I would ask you what happened just before he started to climb the fireplace? How was the very first sip of your tea? I bet you didn't notice, because none of us do. We live in the past, 'I'm glad I saw Amy today, she looked nice. I wonder where she got that top from, she's always so calm with her children. I wish I could be calm like her,' or we live in the future 'I need to get those accounts done, I can't believe I haven't done them yet, if I don't do them, I'll get in trouble, I'll have to do it tonight, but I wanted to do the ironing. I wonder if I'll manage to get both done'. We don't live in the present moment. Unlike when we are in the past or future, the present moment doesn't really have 'words' because it just 'is'. However, I will try to put it into words as follows with the example of drinking a cup of tea: 'I feel the mug in my hands, it feels heavy, my hands warm up around the mug, I feel the ceramic mug against my lower lip, the steam from the tea surrounds my face, my face feels moist, the tea washes

into my mouth, it is warm, my tongue moves in response….'
And so on. Being in the present moment is slow. It is non-judgmental. It is calming. It is blooming difficult, because our over-evolved brains are so good at planning, preparing, analysing and thinking. Our brain defaults immediately to either the future or the past as soon as we let it, and before we know it, we're worrying once more about not being as good as Amy, or about how much work we have to do. So mindfulness takes practice, but it is worth it because it creates calm in an otherwise hectic brain.

Here is the beginner's guide to practising mindfulness. Begin by doing it at the same time each day. This could be as you drop off to sleep at night. It could be as you take a shower. It could be each time you stop at traffic lights. It could be the first sip of your cup of tea. Although Buddhist monks practise mindfulness for hours and hours each day, you can do this for just one minute each day. For the sake of illustration, let us take the example of the shower. Here is a step-by-step guide. Remember that this is difficult, so don't expect miracles straight away.

a. As you get in the shower, make a conscious decision to practise mindfulness for one minute.
b. Take in a deep breath, and breathe out for an even longer breath. Do this twice.
c. As you stand under the water, stop doing anything. Do not begin to wash. Let your arms drop by your side. Put your face under the water (or in a position that feels nice).
d. Notice what it feels like as you stand there. Just stand under the shower. Just stand there. This is your challenge. Just stand there. As you stand there, notice what that feels like. Pay attention to the water

on your skin. Notice the sensation on your skin. Notice how your face feels, notice how your feet feel, notice what you can hear, notice the sensation on your eyelids, notice your heartbeat, and so on. Notice that it feels lovely. Honestly, it will feel *lovely*.

e. Every time your mind goes into default mode, and tries to think about other things, try to notice that this has happened.

f. Then, bring it back to what it feels like to stand under that water.

g. Repeat steps e and f for about a minute.

h. After a minute you will be amazed at how long that minute of your life was, and how much calmer you feel. You have managed to slow your life down a little. Well done.

4. Practising gratitude

Feeling grateful for things, and showing gratitude, has been shown to have emotional benefits. It is also something that can be worked on, rehearsed and practised, until your mind does it automatically. Spending time each day to make a conscious note of the things we are grateful for exercises the part of the brain responsible for good feelings. Traditionally, everyone would have done this at least twice every day in the form of saying 'Grace' before meals and prayer at the end of the day. However, with this daily habit no longer institutionalised in a religious form, we need to find other ways to find gratitude on a daily basis. Affirmations are one way of doing this. 'I am grateful for my physical health, I am grateful that I can do yoga each week' and so on. Diary writing is another. Get into the habit of writing down at the end of the day two things that you are grateful for: 'I am grateful that I got to go to the park, I am grateful that I wasn't in an office all day'. Find habitual times each day to remind yourself of what you are grateful for (before eating, before sleeping, in the shower). Try it for a week and you will want to carry on doing it, because it feels so rewarding.

5. Everyday acts of kindness

Practising being kind has also been shown to light up the parts of the brain associated with good feelings (Robin Youngson). Making a conscious decision to do something for someone that you didn't need to do, on a daily basis, is associated with positive mood and emotional health. There has been an explosion of interest in the benefits of compassion towards yourself and others, in lifting mood and creating positivity. To get into a regular habit of showing little acts of kindness, you just need to make a conscious decision to do so, each day, no matter how big or small. For example, giving to charity, making a cup of tea for someone, giving someone a compliment, buying someone a surprise gift 'just because'. You'll notice that you want to smile, and that nice feeling inside you is reward in itself.

6. Exercise and movement

There is a great deal of evidence to suggest that regular exercise can protect you from developing depression. It is also used as a treatment in its own right. While the physiology is complicated, it seems to be the case that exercise releases 'feel good' hormones such as endorphins, but also that exercise leads the body to produce anti-inflammatory substances, which have been associated with the onset of depression in some people. Intuitively, it also makes sense that if you are feeling angry and frustrated, then it helps to release some of that pent-up energy in the form of exercise. I know it does me the world of good! If you'd like to increase your exercise levels, you need to pick carefully. Many people begin with great intentions, only to find that the habit dwindles after a few weeks or months. Just ask any gym what their attendance rates are in January, and then what they look like in March! It helps to find something that you can get so lost in that you do not notice the passing of time. Team sports are a great way to distract yourself from the fact that you are exercising, unlike gym classes, where you can find the hour goes by quite slowly. Dancing is another great way to exercise without really noticing the time go by. Or ice skating? Rollerblading? Badminton? Walking groups? Fencing? Judo? Wii Fit Sport? Mother and baby buggy fit classes? This is a great chance to have a go at something you've always dreamed about but never done. When you've chosen your activity, it really helps to find someone to do it with, as this also increases your chances of keeping it up. As well as structured classes, why not find a way to increase your activity levels during your normal day-to-day life? Run up the stairs instead of walking. When you take your toddler swimming, put them on your back and swim along with them. They'll love it. Use your baby as your dumbbells, and lift him up regularly like weights. It's great fun. When my baby was little, I would regularly push him up a rather steep hill in his buggy, as part of a regular daily one-mile walk. It became a habit, and slowly other mums began to join me, and we were soon known as the 'infantry' in the village. Those walks and talks were very important in terms of helping me to cope with having babies and toddlers, and I know that I was not the only one.

7. Babywearing

If you haven't considered buying a sling or a baby carrier, now might be the time to do so. While research is a little behind on giving us clear proof of benefits on warding off anxiety and depression, the anecdotal evidence and deductive reasoning make it clear. Research has already shown us the following:

- mum's stress levels are reduced by carrying their baby in a sling
- we know that babies will cry less in a sling
- we know that carrying a baby in a sling increases connection and bonding with your baby
- you can get more done in a day because you have two free hands and a quiet baby
- you can release more oxytocin and endorphins, which feel lovely, and they are an antidote to stress hormones.

Essentially, you get a continual hug from your baby (feels lovely), while you get on with things (what a relief), knowing that your baby is happy with you (no need to worry or go in to check on them). Also, you are doing what nature designed us and all other primates to do: hold and carry our babies. I only discovered the amazing benefits of babywearing with my third child. I would put him on my back as soon as he was old enough (about five months in his case) and he would watch me go about my cleaning and cooking, looking over my shoulder, breathing into my ear, as calm and as peaceful as can be. I knew he adored being in there, and I could not only really enjoy his closeness but also get on with my jobs. It was a million miles away from putting him down on a mat with dangling toys and listening out for him, and frantically hoping that he would last long enough for me to wash some potatoes before he would cry out for attention.

8. Tackle selective bias

Have you ever found yourself comparing yourself to someone else, and feeling a little put out that they are calmer, prettier, happier, more successful, better qualified (and so on and so on) than you are? If the answer is no, I find it difficult to believe you, because comparing ourselves to others is human nature. We all do it. The problem is, we make 'thinking errors' while we do this, especially if we are already feeling a bit inadequate. The first thinking error we make, is that we see one person, or one trait, to the exclusion of all others. For example, we tend to compare ourselves with those that are anywhere near close to how we would like to be ourselves. If you are a runner, you will notice how quickly that woman over there is running. You will not notice how relaxed the dog walker seems to be, because that doesn't interest you. If you are a dog walker, you will notice how good her dog is at recall. You will not notice the jogger. You are more likely to notice other women if you are a woman. If you feel fat, you are more likely to notice thin people. Our comparison with others is highly selective. That makes it automatically highly biased, just like the kid who comes home and says to mum '*All* the other children have the branded trainers'. When you ask carefully, you find out that they mean two children out of thirty. While comparing yourself to others can be a great way to emulate those you admire, it is more often a destructive force than a constructive one. It leads to feelings of inadequacy and self-deprecation. This is because you are making judgements based on fantasy. This is the second thinking error. While you look at the thin jogger, you are singling out the one thing that you wish you were, and making that the be all and end all of the other person's life. You are making hasty judgements. You are presuming you know more about the person than you actually do. For example, with the slim jogger, you are presuming that her slimness, and her running, mean that she is more successful and happier than you are. However, you actually know very little about her life. It may be that she is running in a desperate attempt not to self-harm any more. Or she may be running because if she doesn't, her husband will beat her for being lazy. So, when it comes to watching others, be aware that you are probably making two thinking errors: firstly, only noticing those that you envy, and secondly, making huge assumptions about their lives based on very little evidence. So, every time you notice yourself comparing yourself to someone else, have a chuckle at yourself for catching yourself doing something that is in your nature as a human being, and then correct it with some reminder of how well you are doing.

9. Be your best friend

Do you find that you are harsher on yourself than you are on others? If a friend forgets something, do you say to her 'Don't worry, we all forget things sometimes, it's natural'. If you forget something, do you tell yourself 'Crikey, you complete idiot, what is the matter with you?' While it is very common to be harder on ourselves than we are on other people, I want you to know that it isn't okay. This is because you are actually doing yourself harm. Every time you are horrible to yourself, you flood your system with stress hormones. This is supported by research, because we know that self-critics struggle more with almost every form of mental health problem than non-self critics do. So go easy on yourself. Don't beat yourself up about beating yourself up! Here is a six-step plan for learning to ditch the (do-it-yourself) bitch:

a. Notice you're doing it. This is the hardest step! Acknowledge that you are doing it. Acknowledge you are only human.
b. Take a deep breath in, and a much deeper breath out, twice.
c. Visualise someone who loves you, knows you, and wants to help you feel better.

    d. What would they do? Give you a hug? Tell you it's
        okay? Tell you we all make mistakes? Tell you you're
        wonderful just the way you are?

    e. Close your eyes and imagine them doing it. Really
        imagine them doing it.

    f. Notice that you feel a little better. Amazing! You
        deserve to be treated with kindness just as much
        as your friend does. Practise this, and you will get
        better and better at it.

10. Connect with others

You will have heard of the fight or flight system, which is an adrenalin response to stress. However, have you considered that this evolutionary mechanism would work much better for mobile, non-pregnant or breastfeeding adults than for children and for new mothers? You cannot run or fight effectively if you are heavily pregnant or carrying a baby in your arms. There is another system for keeping yourself safe, which can get activated instead, and that is the 'tend and befriend' system. The theory is that people (especially women) can respond to stress by seeking out the company of others, especially friends. It makes sense, because there is safety in numbers. It also makes sense because, as complex human beings, our problems tend to be socially driven rather than caused by predators. So, by turning to our friends in times of trouble, we keep ourselves feeling safe. Physiologically, friends help us switch off our adrenalin system and activate the 'calm and connect' system. When we become new parents, one piece of advice that is repeatedly given and has been for many years, is to 'get together with other people with new babies'. This is so important. Even if you aren't very sociable, or don't do 'chit chat', find a way to connect with someone other than your partner. Even if you are shy, force yourself to a number of coffee groups/breastfeeding groups/baby swim groups/baby yoga groups/library baby sessions and so on, until you find one you like. Then talk to people. You will not be the only one struggling. Open up and share. This could save your mental health. You are a human being who happens to need other human beings to help you feel calm, reassured, and relaxed.

Taking care of your relationship

Research suggests that relationships are more vulnerable in the first few years after having a baby. This makes sense, because having a baby involves a lot of work, a lack of sleep, some stress and a lot of change and adaptation. But then again, so does moving house – and there isn't much research to suggest that moving house leads to marital break-up. So what is going on?

Well, one factor is that for the first time in our fairly equal lives, the mother and the father are going through different experiences. This means less room for empathy (the ability to understand what someone is going through) and more room for envy (a destructive force). Let me elaborate.

When I was getting used to being a new mum, I remember waiting each day for my husband to come home from work. I would clock-watch, counting down the hours, minutes and seconds. He would come in from work, have a baby thrust into his arms, and hear the woes of his beloved wife fall out of her mouth in a diatribe of emotion.

If he so much as went to a shop on the way home, I was full of envy. 'You did what? You strolled through an aisle, with not a care in the world, browsing and thinking, uninterrupted, slowly selecting what you wanted! What I wouldn't give to be able to do that….'

Poor man. I was thrust into a world that I'd never been in before. While I was getting used to it, he was getting used to me.

This 'envy' thing is a big deal, and it hits us when parenthood hits us. It's big because it threatens our relationships. Up until now, a man and his partner have pretty much experienced the same things. Both have had to go to school. Both have had to cope with exams. Both have had to learn to drive. Both have had to forge a career. Both have had to answer to a boss or company. Both have had to work five days a week. Both know what it is like to come home from work, tired and needing some food, a drink and a sit down. We are equal. We come home, we share making the dinner, we share our stories, and we share a cuddle. But when a baby comes along, for the first time men and women's lives diverge. Now we have a woman at home, with a baby, all day. We have a man trying to maintain his previous levels of functioning at work, coming home to chaos. He suddenly needs to take care of his wife and baby, while keeping his boss happy and preserving his own sanity. So, while she envies his trip to the shop (for the baby wipes that were needed), his point of view might be this. 'You did what? You went to a friend's house for a cup of tea? You chatted, and laughed, with not a care in the world! And the house is a tip. You could at least have tidied up a little'.

He doesn't understand the strains of being at home with a baby. He doesn't understand that sometimes, if mum and baby are dressed and have not gone hungry all day, then that is an achievement. This is not his fault. This is society's fault, for painting motherhood as easy and blissful. It is not, if you are on your own in the house. It is incredibly difficult to do alone.

She doesn't understand how tired he really is. How much in need he is of his pre-baby freedom and carefree life. She doesn't understand what it feels like to have a baby thrust at you when what you need is a smile from your loved one. She doesn't understand that he might be worried about her, feeling like a not-good-enough husband, and full of guilt. (Research shows that, on average, men do not express feelings of guilt, but keep it hidden.)

When we don't understand what is going on for the other person, and when our lives suddenly diverge, envy breeds. Envy is a big divider, as there is nothing good or helpful about it. Envy leads to arguments and accusations, and diminishes compassion and empathy.

There is one very simple way to avoid this happening when you have your baby. It has the following advantages:

1. it gives dad bonding time with his baby
2. it increases dad's confidence in parenting
3. it gives mum a much-needed break
4. it gives dad a chance to develop his own parenting style, his way
5. it reduces the misunderstanding and envy that can arise
6. it increases mutual respect and gratitude towards each other

Have you worked out what it is yet? Just this: Make sure daddy and baby are alone together on a regular basis.

You can begin with just an hour a week. Mums, make sure you go out of the house, leaving him alone with his baby. Then, as the baby becomes less dependent on your breast, you can stretch this to more time away, when you go shopping, or to the spa, or for a haircut, or skydiving. Whatever. It will do you the power of good. It will do his confidence the power of good. And he will begin to understand that being with a baby is a full-time job, and why the house is a tip.

As a mum, you might struggle with this (your mothering hormones are protective and you want to be around all the time). As a dad, you might struggle ('What if baby needs a feed, or I can't settle her'), but the outcome will be fantastic. As a dad, you will begin to feel proud of your parenting ability ('Hey, I can do this'), you will bond more strongly with your little one ('She smiled at me'). As your confidence increases, your respect and empathy for your wife and what she does at home will too. As you understand her situation more, and as your confidence increases, you will naturally help out more in the home. This will reduce the chances of her developing postnatal depression, and that, in turn, will reduce the chances of you developing postnatal depression.

Building in help and support

If you really take on board what I wrote about in the first chapter, you will realise that bringing up a baby is not a job for one woman in a house. It takes a village. You will drop the idea that you 'should' be able to do it, and you will take your needs seriously so that you can express joy and relaxation with your children rather than frustration or indifference.

This is what Suzanne did. She realised that she would need some help, because her husband worked long hours and her family lived abroad. So while she was pregnant with her second baby, she and her husband Rob made the decision to hire an au pair. She said, 'I did not want to get run down myself, with all of the sleepless nights to come. We decided to use an agency to help us hire our first ever au pair and it was a seamless process from start to finish! We offered the wonderful Sarah the job and she arrived one month before our son Jake was born… When Jake came along, I honestly think I wouldn't have made it without Sarah. Sarah was there with me and the two little ones, day in and day out, keeping us all sane. I never looked back on our decision. I know that I had some 'raised eyebrows' from different people. "You mean you have a nanny and you are not going back to work? Why do you need a nanny if you are a stay-at-home mom? Most mothers with live-in au pairs go back to work, you know. Just put them in nursery.' Hearing these comments from people was hard, I felt like I was somehow *weaker* than other mothers. I felt like people would think that I was spoiled and lazy. I questioned our decision as a family. Rob was very supportive and reassured me that in both our hearts, we knew that for our family, this was 100 per cent what we needed. I had to just stay true to my decision and know in my heart that having an au pair saved my sanity and my marriage. It is not always perfect. I think that Rob would sometimes think that because I had the au pair with me I should not have any down/difficult days, but of course you do (just a lot less!). It is a wonderful experience – and to be honest, the au pair system is not overly expensive… when you look at the cost of childcare in nurseries or a babysitter's hourly rate. Even if it was expensive… can you put a price on your sanity? The welfare of your kids? These are priceless!'

Writing a postnatal care plan

How much time and effort have you put into preparing for birth? You may have attended some antenatal classes. You may have investigated and studied pain-relief options. You may have written a birth plan, and given careful thought to what you do and don't want on the day. You may have carefully thought through how you're going to make sure your partner can be there, and who else you may want with you. You may have selected the foods you may want to eat on the day, and made sure your partner knows, so that he can best look after you during your labour. You may have talked it through with your midwife, and so on. You might even have booked a doula. You have put time and effort into making sure that you are looked after on the day, because you know that others will be there to look after you, and that you need that careful attention.

How much time and effort did you put into your wedding day (if you've ever had one, that is)? Many months, lots of money, and plenty of help from friends and professionals alike, no doubt. Even if you had a low-key affair, I bet you did a fair amount of planning.

How much time and effort did you put into planning your last holiday? The hours on the internet, checking for recommendations from friends, planning what you are going to buy to take with you, getting the correct suitcase, making checks with the airline, going shopping for the extras, buying a new pair of sandals, losing weight before you go, getting a spray tan and bikini wax, and so on. The planning and preparing helps you to enjoy your holiday even more.

But how much time and effort have you put into preparing for your first few weeks with a baby? Think about that. How much time and effort have you put into preparing for the first few weeks with your baby?

This is a very special time. This is the time when you are going to fall in love with your baby. This is the time when you are going to grow in confidence. This is the time when you are going to feel closer to your partner. This is the time when you are going to slow right down, cherish togetherness, cry, love and laugh together as you get things wrong, get things right, and learn not to care too much about either. This is the start of the rest of your time as a mother and father. Get the beginning right, and the rest will be easier. Sarah Buckley is a GP specialising in pregnancy and motherhood. Her advice for the postnatal period is to 'Stay in your bedroom for at least a day, stay in your pyjamas for at least a week, stay at home for at least a month. Personally, I think we all deserve our traditional six weeks of nurturing after having a baby'.

My advice is to write a 'baby-moon' plan together. The

term baby-moon has been hijacked, to mean a final holiday before your baby is born. But this makes no sense to me. A honeymoon is when you get to spend special time alone with your new spouse, to get to know each other deeply, and to celebrate your love (in days of old, it was also your first chance to cement your sexual relationship too). A baby-moon is when you get to spend special time alone with your new baby, cement breastfeeding, to get to know each other deeply, and to celebrate your love. Here are some tips for you when planning for your baby-moon.

Plan to stay in bed for a very long time. Maybe buy some lovely breastfeeding-friendly pyjamas – make that two or three sets.

Plan to breastfeed

Research shows us that breastfeeding mothers have lower rates of depression than mothers who don't breastfeed. This makes sense, because when we breastfeed, we release the calming and loving hormone oxytocin. The calming effects help us go back to sleep more easily in the middle of the night after a feed, and generally keep us more chilled and loved-up. It is a pleasure to feed, and sometimes is the only peaceful moment that a new mum gets.

In our culture, the whole issue of breastfeeding has become a bit of a nightmare, with a lot of negativity, pressure and stress surrounding it. If you dearly want to breastfeed, you might need to give this some careful planning if it is something close to your heart (excuse the pun). Prepare by watching lots of videos and photos of other people breastfeeding during your pregnancy. This is a form of mental rehearsal, which is as powerful as actual rehearsal. Speak to people who have done it, and ask them what they enjoyed about it, so that you can begin to think about it in a positive, relaxed way. You might choose to go to a breastfeeding class to learn how wonderfully the whole system works. I would also suggest you plan to get a lactation consultant to your house or the hospital in those early days to help you get on the right track by boosting your confidence that all is going well. If, in spite of all your efforts, you end up going to the bottle, do not blame yourself. This is just adding salt to the wound, and is about as logical as blaming yourself because you have contracted an ulcer. Nature is driving this one, not you. However, even if you don't blame yourself, you may still be left with disappointment and grief for not having had what you so dearly wanted. Allow yourself to grieve, in a self-compassionate way, which will help you to move forward and reap the many rewards that are still open to you.

Vitamins and herbs for recovery

Think about which 'tonics' you usually take to help you feel your best. Buy in your favourite. Look up the benefits of placental encapsulation for example, which is said to be a powerful way to restore vitamins, nutrients and hormonal balance quickly and effectively.

Food

How are you going to eat? You want healthy, easy, enjoyable food. It's not just about having enough pre-prepared frozen food in the freezer. It's also about your snacks, your lunches and your breakfasts. Do not presume that you will have time to put a sandwich together, because you might not. Do not presume that you'll be happy grabbing a banana, because this is a special time that you can never have back again. (Many women vividly remember what they ate around the 'three-day blues' period. It has a special place in their heart.) Food matters. So pre-order your favourite foods for delivery. Include champagne and caviar if that's what you like. My goodness, you deserve some special treatment. You've just made a baby! Ask your friends to make you the dish that you've always loved of theirs, instead of bringing a baby present. Plan in at least one evening for your favourite takeaway, and treat yourselves.

Health care

Think about what helps you feel good when you are a little under the weather. Do you reach for herbal remedies? Homeopathic ones? Your favourite blanket? Do you drink lots? Sleep lots? Do you take yourself to bed? Play some favourite music? Do puzzles? Watch films from your childhood? Whatever it is for you, build it into your baby-moon plan.

Entertainment

If your plan is to stay in bed for most of your baby-moon, you might want to consider some top TV entertainment. Get in your favourite films, favourite dramas and shows, box sets and so on. It needs to be things that are instantly interruptible, because everything in your life will need to be instantly interruptible for the foreseeable future. I would also suggest you plan to stop using Facebook for a while, as it can exacerbate your 'Fear of Missing Out (FOMO)'. As a new parent, you are adapting to the fact that your freedom is curtailed now that you have a baby, and Facebook can make that feeling worse. Music is a wonderful mood enhancer, so make sure you have your favourite music lined up on your device. Also, be sure to include relaxing and calming music, to enhance peace, falling in love with your baby, joy, connection and contentment.

Visitors

Have a plan for managing visitors. You will probably want

visitors, because you want to show off your baby. By all means, enjoy the attention. However, you might find that you don't like passing your baby around. If so, find a way to ensure that doesn't happen. Practising saying 'he gets very fussy when passed around, so I'm going to hold on to him for now'. If you do want people to have the baby so that you can take a break, then ask them if they'd mind holding your baby for a while. They will probably be delighted!

Also, you might find that you get tired very easily, and visitors are staying too long or coming too often. Once again, find a way to deal with this together. Make sure your partner knows, so that he can help to limit the stress. He might even be able to say 'You need to go up and rest now. You go up, and I'll bring you a sandwich'. Whether or not he was going to bring you a sandwich, it should be enough to encourage your visitors to take their leave. It's really important that you do this together, because we are all notoriously bad at following our own advice. But if someone is there telling you to rest, it makes it more likely that you will.

Housework

This one is really important, because midwives, friends and health visitors will tell you to 'leave the housework, it'll wait'. However, I disagree. If you leave the housework, you will soon be sitting in your own dirt, and not even animals like to have to do that. If you get stressed when the house is messy, this is especially important. So find a way to manage the housework. You will need to drop your standards (with parenting, almost every standard you've ever held will need to be dropped to some extent), but you will also need to pre-plan how to manage the housework. You may decide that your partner will do the tidying and cleaning, but remember that tidying and cleaning is quite a big ask when he also needs to help take care of baby, feed you, sleep himself, and take care of his own needs as well as yours. Book a cleaner *more often* than you would have done before. And once again, don't be afraid to ask visitors to help.

People power

Plan who you are going to recruit for their expertise. This is about nurturing yourself, and reducing your stress. There is a wide array of wonderful people that you can decide to enlist, from cleaners to chefs, to masseurs, breastfeeding specialists, dog walkers, ironing people, gardeners, beauty therapists, hairdressers, counsellors, Reiki therapists and postnatal doulas. (Look up postnatal doulas. One might become your guardian angel; they are experts at all the above and very reasonably priced.) If you are going to view becoming a parent as special, like a holiday or a honeymoon or a wedding, then spend some money on pampering yourself. You can do holidays, weddings and honeymoons again, but you can never do a baby-moon again.

The two of you might even want to think about how the two of you will relate to each other during this special time. As well as thinking about the practical stuff, like how the jobs will pan out, how much support dad will give to make sure mum rests, whether dad will stay in, or pop out for a drink with his friends, who will change nappies and so on, you might want to think about how you are going to relate to each other. Things like keeping some physical contact going (non-sexual kisses, hugs, eye contact), arranging time for the two of you to watch some TV you both like or share a takeaway, sharing a compliment a day, and sorting out (tiny amounts of) time to talk. Don't make this too much of a biggie, because you might not have the energy to talk or hug. But in a way, that is why I'm suggesting it. Acknowledge that there won't be much time for this, but also acknowledge that you can support each other and stay connected to some extent.

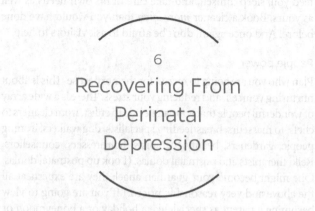

6

Recovering From Perinatal Depression

I am a psychologist. However, I don't think the answer to finding a solution to perinatal depression is in our individual psychology. To think that is to risk blaming the sufferer. I think it is primarily cultural. We need a culture that celebrates and reveres parenthood. A culture that believes women are to be admired, listened to, respected, trusted and celebrated, beyond their sexual allure and into their maternal magic. When she becomes pregnant, we want a woman to feel special. And yet, we have an epidemic of scared women.

In pregnancy, women are frightened of antenatal screening tests, frightened of what they eat, frightened of taking antidepressants, frightened of being stressed. At the birth, they are scared that they will be made to lie on their backs in labour, that they won't be listened to by midwives, that they will have a catalogue of interventions they don't need, or that their bodies will malfunction. After the birth, they are scared that if they cuddle their babies they will kill them and that if the room is too hot, their babies will die. They are scared if they don't breastfeed, scared if they don't sing daily to their baby, scared that they won't lose their baby weight, and scared that they'll get depression. The list is endless. This should not be happening! It is a minor disaster in my eyes. You only need to look at the science, to see that this needs to change. To quote Michel Odent, 'When you meet a pregnant woman, it is your duty to protect her emotional state'. And yet, what happens when we meet a pregnant woman? We tell her our birth horror story. This is not okay, on any level, and it is a symptom of lack of care for and understanding of pregnant women in our society. Research is showing us that this applies to a new mother too. Our duty is to protect her emotional state. We need to take care of her, just as many cultures have in the past and continue to do.

And this isn't just about the mother. We need a culture that puts babies and children first, by prioritising their needs, such as ensuring parents are supported, helping them to feel confident and relaxed during pregnancy, birth and breastfeeding. Let's face it, we are still in a culture which views feeding little babies at the breast as something that needs hiding! That is completely crazy, but because we are in it, we can't actually comprehend how utterly screwed up it is.

And finally, we need a culture that puts fathers at the centre of family life emotionally, allowing them to express their needs and wishes too. Their role needs to be clearer. We expect them to be at the birth, but without any proper preparation. We expect them to become fathers, while the workplace ignores this tremendous transition in their lives. My friend told me this morning that her partner had a business meeting at 7am yesterday. She thought nothing of it. I thought, 'It's a good job he hasn't got little children or a new baby. That is not a father-friendly time to do business'.

So the solution is in our culture. Our culture is changing

rather rapidly, for the better. But the transition process is a rather bumpy ride. And you haven't got time to wait for culture to change. So you need to Do It Yourself for the time being.

The three DIY steps you need to take if you think you might have depression

If someone else tells you that they think you are struggling, or that you could do with some help, or that they think you might have postnatal depression, please listen to them. As much as it might offend you, they are probably right. Sometimes, when you are in the thick of it, you are too busy treading water to see what others can see, or to see how bad it is.

If others can't see it, but you know that you're not well, or happy, or think you might have postnatal depression, or post-traumatic stress disorder, or perinatal OCD, then please listen to yourself. You matter. And your baby will only be little for a short while, so sort it out now, rather than waiting. It is sortable, I promise. Take it seriously. If you had been diagnosed with flu, you wouldn't just carry on regardless. You would help yourself get better. It is the same with depression. Help yourself to get better. There are three steps that encompass all the many ways of getting better that are out there. They are:

1. Tell people
2. Accept offers of help
3. Ask for help

Anyhow, anyway, anybody. Get some help. The first step is telling people how you feel. Tell your GP. Tell your health visitor. Tell your partner. Tell your mother. Tell your friend. Tell your employer. You might get great responses, you might not. Don't rely on people being lovely all the time because they might not be. Your GP might just comment that all mums are tired. Don't be put off, try again and again, and tell someone else. You are looking for the one lovely response that is out there for you.

If you find it difficult to tell people, it is quite likely that you are experiencing some shame about how you feel. Shame is a common and ugly side-kick to depression. It is your depression fooling you, and telling you that you have something to hide, because you are not as good as others. The problem is, that because you hide it you never realise that there are plenty of other people out there, just like you, who feel the same. They are lovely, down-to-earth, successful people, who also happen to be depressed, and believe they aren't as good as others. How can that be? It is because the depression is lying to them too. It's what depression does to us. If you take on board what this book is telling you, there is nothing wrong with you and it is not your fault. Up to 50 per cent of women go through it at some point in their lives, and up to 25 per cent of women have depression around the time that their baby is born. When you tell people, you take your first step to getting better.

Health professionals are there to help you. It is their job. If you decide to tell your GP, health visitor or midwife that you are struggling, or worried, they may ask you to fill out a questionnaire designed to help them decide whether or not you need a referral for help for perinatal depression. This screening questionnaire is known as the Edinburgh Postnatal Depression Scale (EPNS). If you are ever asked to fill out this questionnaire, I would urge you to be honest about your answers. The health professionals are there to help, and because they can't 'see' depression, they can only hear it from you. If you don't like the person who is asking you to fill out the form, or you don't want to open up to them, it is still worth being honest on the questionnaire, because it will prompt a referral to someone who can help. Depending on where you live, you might be asked to fill it out as a matter of routine assessment, regardless of whether or not you seem depressed.

The second step is allowing people to help you. If the GP is suggesting antidepressants, give them a go. If your mother is offering to clean your house on Thursdays, say yes. If your partner is offering to have the baby on his own, let him. If your boss wants to pay for membership to a gym, take it up. If your friend is offering to make you a club sandwich, say yes please. If your neighbour pays you a compliment, accept it. There is no room for misguided 'pride' or comments such as 'I should be able to manage'. You are not well, and you need some help temporarily. Take it seriously. It is not your fault. It is nature's way of telling you that you aren't getting something that you need – be that support, rest, or any of the basic emotional needs that were outlined in Chapter 2. So, as soon as help is offered, take it. Remember the adage that 'it takes a village to raise a baby' and remind yourself that babies thrive with the love and support of their village. Not just one exhausted mother.

The third step is help yourself. Be kind to yourself, allow yourself loads of slack, and take care of yourself. This might mean that you don't have the option of waiting for an offer of help, if it isn't forthcoming, and you need to ask for it. This can be a difficult but important step. As Janine put it, 'If you do not have a good support network, it's easy to get sucked down. Nobody understands and nobody offers what you really crave, which for me was a cuddle and someone to give me just an hour out from time to time'. Thus, sometimes, the only way to mobilise support is to be clear about what you want, and ask. 'I want a cuddle. Tell me you love me, and it's going to be okay.' (This might not be best done with your GP, to be fair!). Or 'Please take the baby out of the house for an hour.' This may be completely alien to you, but here is the start of your learning curve. Ask for help and allow others to help you. If you were running a business, you wouldn't expect to do everything yourself, you would delegate to make your job manageable. This is the same. If you don't have family or friends around, find other ways of getting help. For my third baby, I paid for a childminder for a morning a week, to give me some time to myself. Hire a postnatal doula. They are trained in how to help new mothers thrive – they will clean the house, listen to you, take toddlers out – whatever you both feel you need. They are not expensive. Get a cleaner, an ironing person, a childminder. For my second baby, I arranged with my partner that I would leave the house every Saturday morning for a cycle ride into town to look in shop windows for a couple of hours. I can honestly say it saved my sanity. It 'refuelled' me emotionally for the week ahead.

The following suggestions were put forward by readers of *Juno* magazine, for someone who was suffering with post-natal depression, and had asked for advice. Sufferers and experts alike would agree with them.

'Running! I found following the Couch to 5k running programme really helped. It combated my stress, got me out the house and helped me feel like I was doing something for myself.'

'Online post-natal support groups, Cognitive Behavioural Therapy (CBT), counselling and meditation.'

'Counselling has really helped me and just getting out for a walk to the local post office or park. Cognitive therapy, and try not to be too hard on yourself. Be kind to yourself. Sending hugs.'

'CBT. Be easy on yourself. Lower your expectations of yourself. Be honest with people – let them know how you feel. Get out of the house as much as possible.'

'Exercise outside is a wonderful cure. Find a Buggyfit class or something similar so baby can fit in with you. It's easier to keep going week on week if you know there are others to talk to over a cuppa afterwards!'

'Exercise. Both pulse-raising stuff and more gentle yoga.'

'Birth art helped me so much. It isn't just for birth and pregnancy.'

'I put my daughter into nursery one morning a week. It gave me time to shower, drink a cuppa… have a wee etc. uninterrupted, just for a few hours a week. It really helped! And about five months later she stopped going, as I was feeling stronger. Don't give yourself a hard time – you're doing the hardest job in the world.'

Support groups

There is a burgeoning amount of support available to you out there. There are good organisations that provide information, online support and 24-hour telephone support. There are also Facebook and Twitter groups which can connect you with other sufferers, or other people who have recovered. Sometimes, just having a closed group that you can 'offload' to can make a difference, especially when people reply. This can ease the sense of isolation, and the sense that no one understands. They do. There are many people out there who are going through the same thing as you, and you can reach out to them.

Daily relaxation audio clips

Depression puts your mind and body into a state of constant stress, so you feel unsafe, exhausted and unhappy. The first thing I do when I meet a depressed person for therapy, is help her to relax. Your mind needs a break. A relaxation CD is an easy way to 'breathe' and get some air. It puts the body into a restorative, oxytocin and endorphin-rich state, giving you relief from your usual tense and stressed state. There are plenty to choose from. Some are specifically designed for pregnancy and parenthood. But any relaxation download will help. Find one that you like and listen to it when you go to bed. Don't worry if it doesn't seem to relax you, or if you go straight to sleep and feel like you've missed it. The beauty of relaxation tracks is that there are no side-effects, they almost always do some good, and they get better the more you listen to them. What have you got to lose?

Therapy and counselling for perinatal depression

There are a number of therapy interventions on offer, and I will cover them in order of their complexity or sophistication.

First of all, counselling gives you something that is very difficult to get in life, but that feels very precious. That 'something' is this: someone *listening*, exclusively and actively to you, for more than ten minutes at a time. Having space to talk and think and reflect on how you're feeling is pretty special. Having permission to put yourself first, to cry if you want to without guilt, to get angry if you want to without repercussion, to say things that you've been thinking but didn't dare say, to make sense of the things that do matter and the things that don't matter so much, can be wonderful. And the great thing about counselling is that the person listening to you is *on your side*. They understand that underneath all the tears and the confusion is someone amazing who is trying her best, and will get through this. They hold your self-esteem and your hope for you, while you muddle your way through, trying to find it for yourself. Good counselling is worth its weight in gold.

If you go to your GP, you might be offered counselling via their in-house counsellor. Or you might be offered Cognitive Behavioural Therapy (CBT) via a government scheme called

IAPT (Improving Access to Psychological Therapies). CBT includes the benefits of counselling, as someone listens to you and gives you space to express what is going on for you. But CBT is also more structured, and specific time will be put aside to help you understand the 'thinking patterns' that might be making life harder for you. These include those we have already spoken about, such as 'selective bias' or believing that you'll never get better, or that others will be better off without you. The way we think can make us feel worse, and when we are depressed our thinking becomes even more negative. So CBT aims to address that imbalance, and get you back in touch with more realistic ways of thinking, such as 'I'm a good enough mother', or 'I want to go a little easier on myself because that will help'.

A third form of help, available on the NHS, is a special perinatal mental health service, although not all areas have this yet. A specialist perinatal mental health team will include professionals who exclusively work with parents around the time that they have their baby. This is a tertiary service, which means that it is designed for people for whom counselling and CBT isn't quite enough, and they need another level of care. These teams usually have specialist mental health midwives and clinical psychologists in them. Speaking as a clinical psychologist myself, their level of training and expertise is excellent. And I'm not just saying that. It takes at least six years to train as a clinical psychologist.

If you go to your GP and tell them that you are struggling with what you think is perinatal depression, be aware that you will probably be offered medication. Many people find this very beneficial. Antidepressants take about three weeks to take effect. Once they do, they can make a dramatic difference to your mood. As your mood lifts, you might find it easier to put into practice all the other forms of self-help that this book covers, and get yourself into a much better place within weeks or months.

Whether or not you decide to use the antidepressants, the option of a 'talking therapy' should still be on the table. In fact, research suggests that a combination of antidepressants and talking treatment is the most effective combination, in terms of staying well after you've stopped the treatment. If medication isn't for you, be clear with your GP that you decline the drugs, but that you still want help. You are completely within your rights to do this, especially as the medication can have side-effects, be unpleasant to withdraw from, and seems to be only as effective as placebo for mild to moderate depression. If you know that you want some form of talking treatment, say this to your GP. If you find that difficult, take someone with you to the consultation, who can support you in telling the GP what you would like.

While the NHS is there to help you, you may not always click with the counsellor attached to your GP, or your CBT therapist or psychologist. Also, the NHS often operates a waiting list, and the sooner you can get help, the better. For that reason, you might want to source your own counselling or therapy. Go online and have a browse. Check credentials, give them a ring, and get a feel for whether they sound like they could help. If you're not sure, meet them anyway and give it a go. It can take some determination and courage, but it might end up making all the difference to how you feel and how quickly you recover.

Clean up your act

If you are suffering from depression, you need to take care of your mind and body. You cannot expect an engine to run well on dirty fuel. And your mind and body will not run well on junk food, no exercise and no sleep. So, first watch what you eat. Eat healthily; cut out the caffeine, crisps and biscuits. Second, build some exercise into your day, even if you start with just a short walk each day. Third, practise some sleep hygiene. This means taking yourself to bed properly, rather than kipping on the sofa. You can put an eye mask on to help you get the most from the time that you do have to sleep. Cutting out caffeine will also help. Turn your phone off before you intend to sleep (without checking it first). Download a ten-minute relaxation or meditation app to do each day. Let others know that you are sleeping, to reduce the chances of being disturbed unnecessarily.

Do your daily A & E

When we are depressed, we often feel worthless and we find it difficult to enjoy things. As a result, things that make us feel like we have achieved something (our A) and things that we enjoy (our E) fall by the wayside. This is a problem, because in order to boost our mood, we need to gain a sense of achievement and we need to enjoy things (our A & E). Research has shown that if we *force* ourselves to do one thing each day which constitutes an achievement, and one thing each day which is enjoyable, we can slowly shift our mood over time. I say 'force' because it can be quite an effort when we are depressed. A therapist will help you with this, but if you are doing it on your own maybe you can recruit a family member to help. Here's how you do it.

1. Think of one thing that you would like to achieve in the day. Keep it small. Don't imagine that you are better, and write down something you could easily have done before you got depressed. Write something in proportion to how you feel at the moment. So, keep it small. It might be to go out to

the shop, or do a wash load, or phone the bank. It might be to get dressed. Write it down.

2. Think of one thing that you used to enjoy. I say *used* to enjoy, because it might be that the depression is stopping you from enjoying anything at the moment. It might be 'read a magazine' or 'watch a soap opera' or 'do a jigsaw' or 'take a bath'. Write it down.

3. Do this every day, and make sure you actually fulfil it. Don't worry how you *feel* while you're doing it. Just make sure you do it.

4. When you have done it, give yourself a pat on the back, and plan the next day's A & E. Always keep it small and manageable, because I want you to always succeed.

Identify your needs and find a way to meet them

As mentioned in Chapter 2, we all have a basic need for security, attention, control, emotional connectedness, community, privacy, status, competence and meaning. If any one of these is not being met, you will struggle emotionally. When my babies were little, I very much needed extra community and privacy. Making sure that these needs were met made an enormous difference to my mental health. It will to yours too. The need for privacy, or 'me-time', is a very common need in new mothers. Take this need seriously, and find time for you. If dad isn't around, hire a babysitter for two hours a week. Go to a coffee bar, a nail bar, go swimming, go paragliding for all I care. Just do something for you, on a regular basis. Never forget how important you are, and how much you matter now that you are a mum. If this is difficult for you because your baby is young, or you are attachment parenting, or feeding on demand, then start with 20 minutes at a time and build it up. Babies are built to be cared for by a number of caretakers at any one time. Having said that, it might be wise to avoid any drastic separations from your baby at the two peak attachment periods. These are usually at around nine months (can be as early as six months, when they begin to be wary of strangers) and at around two years. You will probably notice them, because your baby will become more clingy than usual.

What about treatment for post-traumatic stress disorder?

As mentioned earlier, there are effective treatments available for trauma. You probably find that hard to believe, because it feels so ingrained in you now. I have been treating trauma for over 20 years, with an enormous amount of success. It is treatable. I promise you. Don't fight on your own, because some people spend all their lives traumatised, until they receive treatment. War veterans have suffered for decades with PTSD, until a short course of treatment lifts it. And it can really feel like something has been lifted. As one person once said to me, 'It was here – in my forehead – I couldn't get rid of it – always there – always in my way. It has gone. I can't believe it, it has totally gone'. Treatments involve reprocessing the memory from the 'I'm not safe' (threat activated) part of the brain, and laying the memory to rest in the 'it was awful but it's over' part of the brain.

Here are some things you can do to help you to heal from your traumatic birth.

Recruit support

Make sure you reach out to people. Let them look after you. Tell them what is going on for you. If you had broken your leg, you would ask people to help you, and you wouldn't feel bad for telling them all about it.

Remember that you matter too

For too long, our society has thought that it is okay to believe that 'All that matters is a healthy baby'. This is simply not true, because you matter too. Furthermore, you matter more now than you did before your baby's existence, because we want to keep you strong so that you can keep your baby strong.

Remember that you are allowed to feel angry and sad at the same time

You might feel guilty because your beautiful baby is here, alive and well, and all you can do is cry and feel angry about how he got here. This is completely rational, reasonable and understandable. You do not need to feel bad or guilty for this. It is normal to feel grateful and angry or upset at the same time. If I had been mugged in the street, I could feel grateful that I am still alive and that others are supporting me, at the same time as feeling upset and devastated that it happened in the first place.

Find ways of processing the memory, rather than avoiding it

For example, cry when you need to. Tell people what happened in detail. Many people find that writing down what happened in detail is very healing. Focus on how you felt and what you thought at every stage. While you are writing or talking, allow yourself to feel anger, if people treated you badly. Finish your writing with a strong statement about how strong you were to cope with what happened, even if you don't quite believe that. Then, when you have done this, burn it, tear it up, or ceremoniously bury it.

Whatever you do, don't hide it

You have nothing to be ashamed of. This is not your fault. Give your body and mind time and space to recover, by getting help to eat and rest, and by letting people be kind to you. Your smile, your love, your laughter, will come back. Bit by bit. And if, after six months, it still isn't beginning to come back, get more help.

Getting professional help for PTSD

In my experience, the NHS is not always the best place to go for treatment, although this does depend on the services available in your local area. If you go for treatment on the NHS, ask for EMDR (Eye Movement Desensitisation and Reprocessing). Counselling may help you feel better, but research suggests it might not treat the PTSD, so don't settle for the GP counsellor if you really think you have PTSD.

If you decide to try a private therapist, take your time finding someone with relevant training and experience. I use the rewind technique (a hypnotic technique, taught to me by the Human Givens Institute), which seems to be the most effective, quickest, and least distressing treatment. It can work in one session. I also use cognitive behavioural techniques (CBT), which are also 'evidence based' (NHS jargon to say that it has been through rigorous research to demonstrate that it works). Eye Movement Desensitisation and Reprocessing (EMDR) is known to be effective too. A non-evidence-based therapy that I've also heard good things about is the Emotional Freedom Technique (the 'tapping' one). Most hypnotherapists are very effective at lifting trauma, using a number of visualisations and reframing techniques to reprocess the memory.

Please note that I am only recommending the *therapy* in general, not all the *therapists* who say they practise the techniques. Be picky about the therapist, and find one that works for you.

The road to recovery

As outlined above, in cases of PTSD, recovery can be instant. However, with depression, the road to recovery tends to be a little bumpier. Recovering from depression isn't quick and it isn't easy. There will be days when you feel you are back to square one. This is because recovery does not follow a neat graph with a straight line. It doesn't even follow a curvy up and down line. It follows a line of circles, squiggles, and interweaving loops. However, please remember that you will never actually be back to where you were (even if it feels like that sometimes), because you have been learning throughout your journey, and no one can ever take away what you have learnt. Think of the recovery as being like a game of snakes and ladders. There will be some days when you fall down the ladder, but you never get right back to the beginning. You slowly but surely make your way up, even when you think it will never happen. If you ever doubt that you will get better, talk to others who have recovered. They will tell you that they never thought they would get better either. But they did.

Fear of going back there again

Once we have recovered from depression, we can find ourselves feeling frightened of bad feelings, because we get worried that we are going back to that awful state again. Even well people have bad days! Even well people feel anxious, or inadequate, or frustrated to bursting point. When you are better, you will still have all these feelings. These are what make you human, so don't be scared that you are going to get ill again. They do not equal depression. They equal normal everyday life. All of us should be doing our regular 'self-care' regimes, as outlined in Chapter 5, just as we should be exercising regularly. Keep it up, and you will have fewer and fewer bad days.

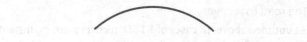

Conclusion

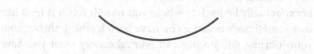

I don't have much to say in conclusion, other than that you have my admiration. Any parent in this day and age has my admiration. Parenting has become a bit of a psychological nightmare with such conflicting advice, and with far too much information out there, and with the loss of the 'village', and the knowing, calming and reassuring elders who have done it all before. I am a believer in scientific understanding, but I think it should be left in the laboratories and the journals. It has no place in your home. Your home is yours and it is where you love, laugh, cry, connect, argue, reconnect, find adventure and find peace. You are resilient and so is your baby. Kick back and watch her grow, because you won't be able to stop it happening, no matter how many mistakes you make as her parent. One day, you'll be looking back and watching her in admiration, aware that she has grown up to be an incredible adult with jobs and friends and everything, in spite of all the mistakes you made and the worrying you did.

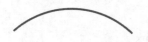

Further Reading and Resources

Books

Steven Biddulph, *Manhood*, Vermilion, 2012

Sarah Buckley, *Gentle Birth, Gentle Mothering*, Celestial Arts, 2009

Michelle Cree, *The Compassionate Mind Approach To Postnatal Depression: Using Compassion Focused Therapy to Enhance Mood, Confidence and Bonding*, Robinson, 2015

Sue Gerhardt, *Why Love Matters: How Affection Shapes a Baby's Brain*, Routledge, 2014

Kerstin Uvnäs Moberg, *The Oxytocin Factor: Tapping the Hormone of Calm, Love and Healing*, Pinter & Martin, 2011

Naomi Stadlen, *What Mothers Do: Especially When it Looks Like Nothing*, Piatkus, 2005

Websites

apni.org

home-start.org.uk

lift-depression.com

maternalocd.org

mind.org.uk

pandasfoundation.org.uk

samaritans.org

time-to-change.org.uk

yourbirthright.co.uk/parents-to-be

Index

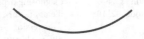